The
Book
of the
Back

Brian Inglis

The Book of the Back

HEARST BOOKS
New York

First published 1978
by Ebury Press
Chestergate House
Vauxhall Bridge Road
London SW1V 1HF

ISBN 0 85223 133 4

Drawings on pages 19, 49, 50, 60, 127, 133,
135, 136, 137: by Chris Evans
Designed by Derek Morrison
Edited by Isabel Sutherland

Filmset and printed in Great Britain by
BAS Printers Limited, Over Wallop, Hampshire
and bound by
Redwood Burn Ltd, Esher, Surrey

Contents

Acknowledgments

In the early stages of research for *The Book of the Back* I received invaluable help from Fiona Pearson, Editorial Manager of *World Medicine*, and from Helene Graham; giving me guidance on where to go to find the required sources, and whom to see (and, on occasion, whom to avoid encountering). Helene also read the typescript, and Fiona the proofs, rescuing me from many errors. John Ebbetts, R. Newman Turner and Ruth West also read and commented upon the typescript; and Bernard Levin found the time to read, and provide characteristic caustic comments upon, the proofs. I am grateful to them all.

I also received good advice and assistance from the organizations listed; from Jock Anderson, Sammy Ball, Ronald Barbor, A. H. Bosman, M. E. Burleigh Carson, J. H. Davidson, Colin Dove, Thomas Dummer, Liz Ferris, Rodney Graham, Stewart Korth, and Terry Moule, all workers in this field; and from many doctors encountered casually, or at meetings, who put forward fruitful ideas and suggested sources of which I would not otherwise have heard.

BRIAN INGLIS

The publishers wish to thank the many people and institutions who have given permission to reproduce the pictures in this book. The Leonardo da Vinci drawings on pages 41 and 43 are reproduced by gracious permission of HM The Queen. We are also indebted to The Wellcome Trustees; the British School of Osteopathy; Robert Jones and Agnes Hunt Orthopaedic Hospital; the Institute of Orthopaedics; the Acupuncture Association and Register Ltd., the Radionic Association; Ashe Laboratories Ltd; Dr Wilfred Barlow, and Arrow Books Ltd for permission to use the cover photograph from his book, *The Alexander Principle*; Churchill Livingstone for permission to use the drawings of James Mennell's manipulative techniques; and Dr Charles Burton of the Sister Kenny Institute, Minneapolis, for allowing us to re-draw the diagram of a TENS device that appeared in his booklet, *Be Good to Your Back*.

Introduction

You stoop down one morning to put on a shoe – or one evening to pull up a weed in the garden – and suddenly something seems to 'give' in the small of your back, and you find yourself in agony, unable to stand upright, barely able to totter to a sofa or your bed. So you decide to call your doctor. What happens next depends on where you live. In many American cities 'your' doctor will simply be a man you know whom you can ring up to ask which specialist to consult; for the old-style family doctor has almost become extinct. But in Europe he survives; and in Britain the General Practitioner flourishes in spite of his grumbles at the National Health Service. He will even, as a rule, come round to your home, if your back is so bad that you feel you cannot get to him.

Whether GP or specialist, his examination and prescription are likely to follow the same course. He will do some tests for joint mobility, and some to locate which movements cause you pain; but unless he finds a symptom requiring immediate attention, which he might come across one time in a hundred similar visits to attend such cases, he will recommend you to rest in whatever position you find least uncomfortable; and prescribe some mild analgesic drug, usually aspirin, as a pain-killer.

Often the rest works. The pain goes away in a few hours, or a few days. But if it does not go away, one or other or both of you will want a second opinion; and as a rule this will entail a visit to a hospital or clinic. There, the tests already done will be repeated, along with others backed by a more elaborate battery of investigative procedures, assisted by radiography and gadgets which actually measure, as distinct simply from estimating, mobility; along with tests of the blood, the urine, the cerebrospinal fluid, the body's phosphates and much else besides.

At the end of it all, however, the chances are that what will be prescribed will not be very different from what the GP advised: basically, rest, to leave nature to promote recovery. You may be provided with additional assistance in the form of a plaster jacket or a surgical corset, or a brace, designed to try to keep the affected vertebrae immobile, while leaving you relatively mobile so that you can return, if you have to, to your job. You may be prescribed physiotherapy, with heat treatment, massage and exercises (though they will often be intended less to speed your recovery than to keep the rest of your muscles in working order). You may be given 'traction' – a procedure involving the application of a pulling force, for example by weights suspended on pulleys above the patient's bed – in the hope that stretching your ligaments and musculature will help; you may have pain-killing injections; or you may have a course of anti-inflammatory drugs – though these have proved so unsuccessful, and on occasions so deplorable in their side-effects, that they are now suspect – which, unfortunately, has not stopped some GPs from continuing to prescribe them. But the chances are that if your backache persists – if it has not been traced to some specific disease, such as an infection or cancer – and you do not have to be up and about, you will be on bed and aspirin, again.

Orthodox medicine, in other words, is short of ideas for dealing with – as distinct from palliating – back pain. This, in spite of the fact that it is one of the commonest disorders of civilization. Precisely how prevalent it is remains difficult to say with any pretensions to accuracy, though there is no shortage of guesses. A few years ago, while *Life* lived, one of its writers claimed that nearly 30,000,000 people went every year in the United States to have their backs 'stretched, straightened, sprayed, heated, cooled, injected, manipulated, massaged or just looked at'. A more cautious recent estimate has put the figure at 17,000,000, of which 2,000,000 are new patients; with 200,000,000 working days being lost as a consequence. In Britain the equivalent figures, according to Dr David Delvin – medical editor of the *General Practitioner*, and author on behalf of the Back Pain Association of *You and Your Back* – are 1,500,000 cases, and 15,000,000 working days lost ('almost certainly', Delvin claims, 'every year one in twenty-five people in Britain goes to the doctor about back pain'). As a cause of lost working days it is fourth in the league, behind bronchitis (and other respiratory disorders), influenza, and heart trouble of various kinds.

8

But from the nature of backache, such figures can at best be a very rough guide. Most estimates include only consultations with members of the medical profession, which inevitably miss out those sufferers who prefer to take their bad backs to medically unqualified practitioners, or to nobody at all. Figures for working days lost through back pain do not include uncertified absenteeism – or housework; if they were added in, they would make a formidable addition. And it has come to be accepted that as well as lumbago, as pain in the lower back is commonly (though rather less commonly than it used to be) described, other types of pain like sciatica – shooting pains in the limbs – which used to be attributed to a 'chill' caught by sitting in draughts or getting drenched in a shower, are in reality 'referred' from the spine. Recently the tendency has also been to re-categorize as 'referred pain' – again referred from the spine – many of the miscellaneous symptoms which used to be labelled rheumatism, arthritis, or fibrositis; more than half of all sickness so labelled, Swedish researchers have claimed, can be traced to some spinal defect, and a follow-up study undertaken for the Industrial Survey Unit of the British Arthritis and Rheumatism Council has provided confirmation, its report pointing to the conclusion that 60 per cent of what has been called rheumatism is, properly speaking, back trouble. The estimates may consequently need to be revised sharply upwards, perhaps putting backache in second place in the working-days-lost table.

As a consequence, the problem has been attracting more attention. In America the emphasis has been on research into the nerve mechanism of pain; in Britain it has been on how to reduce working days lost.

In Britain in 1975 Dr David Owen, Minister of State for Health, criticized the Medical Research Council for devoting too much of its attention and its funds to esoteric complaints, and recommended it instead to support more research into back pain (a point of view he was to reiterate on other occasions while he remained in the Department of Health); and a few months later Len Murray, General Secretary of the Trades Union Congress, urged Unions to pressure employers to take more effective measures to reduce the incidence of backache among manual workers. A Working Group has since been set up by the Department of Health under the Chairmanship of Professor A. L. Cochrane to review the existing provisions for dealing with back pain; to decide on what questions need to be answered in order to improve them; and to advise on the desirability of clinics to provide early treatment and advice on prevention.

An investigation of this kind had been energetically lobbied for by the Back Pain Association, a charity set up to raise funds for research and to promote a better understanding of the causes of back pain, and how to prevent it. Such charities are normally dominated by the medical profession; but the Association had been making no secret of its members' dissatisfaction with orthodoxy, and this is reflected in the evidence it has presented to the Cochrane Committee. It has received 20,000 letters asking for the Association's booklet *You and Your Back*, many of them extremely critical of their doctors.

> It seems as if there is a lack of a proper approach to diagnosis and treatment. Many GPs and consultants find back pain a chore, and only a small proportion of back troubles are being properly managed . . . Provision for treatment is virtually non-existent in some areas. The delay in getting an appointment for a patient to see a consultant is a major deficiency. In some areas in NW England there is a nine months' wait for non-urgent out-patient departments. . . . Physiotherapy is frequently recommended for any back condition, but facilities generally are totally in-adequate. . . .

and so on. Clearly it is not just a question, as in other disorders, of delays in obtaining treatment: there is little prospect of the treatment being effective even when it is obtained.

It is not, however, necessary to rely on the medical profession for treatment for back pain. If your stay in bed lasts more than a day or two, the chances are that one or more of your visitors will tell you that you are crazy not to go to an osteopath, or chiropractor, or acupuncturist. In this respect, backache is unique among the common disorders. None of the others has such an army of para-medical practitioners waiting in the wings for your custom; an army, furthermore, which enjoys a public image far removed from that of the 'quack' of tradition.

The Book of the Back is primarily a survey of the various alter-natives, orthodox and unorthodox, which are open to you as a backache sufferer – not with a view to promoting any of them, but simply to give some guidance on what the options (and the risks) are. It deals chiefly with backache of the kind doctors used to call 'functional', and now more often describe as 'non-specific': that is, pain which cannot be traced (not, at least, with certainty) to a specific cause – a congenital disease, say, like spina bifida, or a bone infection like TB, or a spinal tumour. Of course it is important that such diseases should be diagnosed; but they represent only a tiny fraction of back cases.

There is a tendency to think of the story of medicine as a record of development from the darkness of primitive superstition to the light of modern science, periodically interrupted by setbacks, but on balance a triumphant progress. Not so with backache. The record here is of explorations of what have turned out to be blind alleys: worse, of refusal to admit that they are blind, and of obstinate perseverance with irrelevant diagnostic procedures and useless, even dangerous, forms of treatment. And this is why it is so desirable to study the historical background; to dispose of the notion that what the doctor orders is likely to be sound, or even safe. History also helps to put the various forms of alternative medicine, as it is now coming to be called, in perspective. It does not, unfortunately, point unerringly to any one form as being the most trustworthy. After reading the typescript of *The Book of the Back*, in fact, a friend of mine suggested that it might well be re-named *Naught for your Comfort*. It offers no nostrums. But it does give pointers; and they may be a help to you in finding what you are looking for, if you should decide to shop around for treatment.

The Medical Heritage

The Medical Heritage

Of all human disorders, backache ought to be among the simplest to track down to its evolutionary origins. As Henry Sigerist remarked in the first volume, published in 1951, of a work which, had he lived to complete it, would have been both a monumental and a wonderfully perceptive history of medicine, only one organ system, that of the bones, 'survives the centuries and millennia'; making it possible to trace diseases of the spine in fossil remains. The great dinosaur in the Natural History Museum in Kensington evidently suffered from arthritis; most of the vertebral disorders known to modern man have been found in fossilized animals and in the skeletons of primitive man, as have almost all known deformations, including spina bifida, in mummies preserved by design, or in skeletons preserved by chance, from early civilizations.

The temptation has consequently been to attribute back disorders to the fact that man has not yet fully adapted to the upright stance which he acquired in the course of his evolution; and to this day, many writers on the subject point to the problems posed because man's spine and its attachments were not designed by nature for the purpose for which he now uses them. But this view was disputed by Sir Arthur Keith, writing half a century ago – and writing with a grace and lucidity now all too rarely found in medical works. Rapid though the switch to standing upright must have been in evolutionary terms, he felt, compelling the invention of all sorts of makeshift devices to keep the various organs of the body in their places, what impressed him was the extraordinarily effective way in which the necessary adaptation had been carried out. So far from being in any way inadequate for the performance of its duties, he suggested, the human spine was a superb piece of anatomical and functional engineering, which could hardly have been bettered if it had been created by design rather than by natural selection; and he described in graphic detail the devices built in to provide the maximum of mobility and flexibility with the maximum of safety. There was no point in blaming the spine, he felt, or the whole nervous and muscular system which it sustains, for what goes wrong with it. If the system becomes disordered, it is through accident, or infection, or misuse.

The earliest recorded treatment

In any case, although the remains of fossilized or mummified man have much to tell us about spinal diseases and infections, they disclose very little about what, if any, treatments were used. There is a brief reference to treatment in the time of the Pharaohs in the 'Edwin Smith Papyrus' recommending rest, and a diet of fresh meat and honey; but it is incomplete. The first reasonably detailed account of the treatment of back disorders dates from the 5th century BC, in the works of Hippocrates. As with Homer, there is no contemporary account of Hippocrates as an individual; the writings, collected a couple of centuries later, may have been taken from a number of sources. But they were to be extremely influential, offering as they did the first calm and clear account of the disorders from which man suffered, and what could be done to ameliorate them.

Nothing very much, Hippocrates admitted, *could* be done, to alter the course of most illnesses, except by giving every assistance possible to the healing force of nature, with rest and an appropriate diet. But he accepted that it might be possible to do something about a spine which had been bent forward, whether by accident, habit, pain, or advancing years; with the aid of traction or succussion – shaking – to force the vertebrae apart, so that they could be maneuvered back into their correct position, by hand or some other means.

The method of traction he favoured involved placing the patient on a board, and tying thongs round his ankles, knees, loins and armpits. The physician 'or some person who is strong, and not uninstructed, should apply the palm of one hand to the hump and then, having laid the other hand upon the former, he should make pressure, gauging whether this force should be applied directly downward, or toward the head, or toward the hips'. The method, Hippocrates insisted, was safe. It was safe, too, for the doctor to put his foot on the bent spine, or even to bounce up and down on it, the better to straighten it out. And hazardous though the method now sounds, similar methods have been reported by anthropologists working with tribal communities, by historians, and by folk-lore enthusiasts collecting material, in many parts of the world; which has prompted the medical historian Dr Eiler Schiötz of Oslo to say that if such methods have been found effective in countries as far apart as Norway, Mexico and the Pacific islands, 'over many, many centuries', the inference is that they must have some validity.

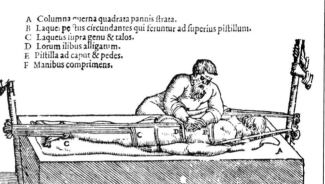

A Columna ◌uerna quadrata pannis ſtrata.
B Laquei pe ſtus circundantes qui feruntur ad ſuperius piſtillum.
C Laqueus ſupra genu & talos.
D Lorum ilibus alligatum.
E Piſtilla ad caput & pedes.
F Manibus comprimens.

A method of traction and sustained pressure recommended in the works of Hippocrates.
Galen, after Hippocrates; Courtesy, The Wellcome Trustees

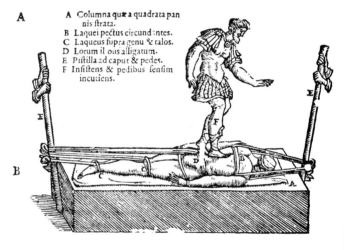

A Columna quæ a quadrata pannis ſtrata.
B Laquei pectus circund intes.
C Laqueus ſupra genu & talos.
D Lorum il ous alligatum.
E Piſtilla ad caput & pedes.
F Inſiſtens & pedibus ſenſim incutiens.

A man standing on the sufferer's back to apply pressure in the course of traction.
Galen, after Hippocrates; Courtesy, The Wellcome Trustees

The alternative, succussion, involved strapping the patient to a ladder, which could be shaken up and down to loosen his vertebrae. Hippocrates was prepared to give credit to the individual who had thought of the idea, 'or any other contrivance which is according to nature'; but so far as he knew, the method had never succeeded in straightening out anybody's bent spine. He was suspicious of it, too, because he had observed that it was 'principally practised by those physicians who seek to astonish the mob – for to them, such things appear wonderful, when they see a man suspended and thrown down, or the like; they always extol such exhibitions and never concern themselves about whether the results of the experiment are good or bad'. The doctors who used the method, in Hippocrates' experience, were not to be trusted. He was unwilling to reject the possibility that the spine might be helped by succussion, if it were properly understood and carried out; but for his part, he would not care to treat cases in this way, because such procedures were generally practised by charlatans.

The birth of orthodoxy

It was the first manifesto for what has since come to be called 'conservative' treatment: and Hippocrates reinforced it with a more forthright attack on those practitioners who claimed they could treat cases of derangement where the spine was bent inwards – say, in an accident. The least displacement of the vertebrae in this way, he argued, compressed or strangled the spinal cord; paralysis and other symptoms were inevitable; and no doctor could hope to intervene successfully – for to do so would require opening up the body, and pulling the spine out, as it were, from within, which could only be done with a corpse.

> Why, therefore, do I write all this? Because certain persons fancy they have cured patients in whom the vertebrae had undergone complete dislocation forward. Some, indeed, suppose that this is the easiest of all these dislocations to be recovered from, and that such cases do not stand in need of reduction, but get well spontaneously. Many are ignorant, and profit by their ignorance, for they obtain credit from those about them.

Hippocrates was anticipating a controversy which has continued to this day. There would have been no accepted distinction in his time between 'luxation' and 'subluxation' – actual dislocation of the

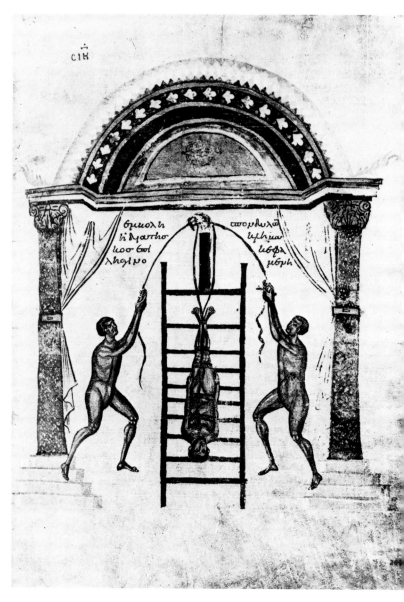

Succussion, another Ancient Greek method of treating backache; the patient was strapped to a ladder which was shaken up and down to loosen his vertebrae.
Apollonius von Kitium: Courtesy, The Wellcome Trustees

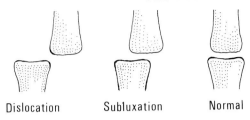

A joint in the normal condition (right), 'subluxated' or slightly displaced (centre) and 'luxated' or dislocated (left). In Hippocrates' time, no clear distinction was generally recognized between slight displacement and actual dislocation.

vertebrae, and slight displacement. He appears to have been attacking the unqualified practitioners, just as they were to be attacked again nearly two and a half millennia later, for doing something which he assumed was anatomically impossible – mending a dislocated spine. But the manipulators, then as now, were presumably concerned less with the anatomy of the spine than with the way it functioned. If it began to function again as a result of manipulation, or any other treatment, that was what mattered – whatever the cause might be. Galen, the Greek physician, agreed. Writing in the 2nd century AD, he speculated that spinal vertebrae could get out of alignment with each other, even when there was no actual dislocation; and in such cases, they could be put right by lining them up again.

It was the conservative method which survived, however: rest, sometimes coupled with traction, applied either manually or with the help of gadgetry. In the 16th century the French surgeon Ambroise Paré employed servants to pull on a strap placed under his patient's arms and shoulders, while others pulled at his feet, to allow Paré to put him in a splint while he was stretched; or, if the neck were the seat of the trouble, he had his servants press on the patient's shoulders while he took the head in his hands, lifted it, and turned it from side to side. But references to such treatment by doctors are rare, for a reason which was only to begin to become clear from a controversy which arose in the 18th century.

The presumptuous bone-setter
According to an article in the *London Magazine* in 1736, the capital had begun to be intrigued 'by the fame of a young woman at Epsom

who, though not very regularly, it is said, has wrought such cures that seem miraculous, in the bone-setting way': cures which earned her – or so it was estimated – around 20 guineas a day, because she was able to do what she did in 'so very quick a manner'. Some London surgeons, irritated by her presumption, had thought to expose her by sending her a man who pretended that his wrist was out of joint: 'she gave it a wrench, which really put it out, and bade him go to the fools who sent him, and get it set again'. Sarah Mapp drew her clients from society – even, it was believed, from royalty. But this was unusual. Most bone-setters came from the artisan class and worked within it; their activities rarely attracted the attention of physicians.

That somebody who had dislocated a joint should go to the local bone-setter, rather than to a doctor, was not surpising. Reducing dislocations was a craft most easily learned by apprenticeship, and required no education. Physicians, who at that time considered themselves to be the only real doctors, appear to have regarded it as beneath their dignity – much as they regarded tooth-pulling or, for that matter, surgery of any kind. And the surgeons, battling for respectability, were increasingly coming to think of themselves as practitioners of what is now taken to be their chief, and indeed only, function: the opening up (or in the case of wounds, the closing up) of the body. As for the apothecaries, forerunners of the present day general practitioner, they usually grew up in or around where they were to practise, and they learned their craft by apprenticeship, picking up manipulation to reduce fractures or dislocations as part of their training. They were not regarded as doctors – not, at least, by the physicians and surgeons. What they did was their own affair.

Towards the end of the 18th century, though, a new medical specialty began to develop: orthopedics. The term was first used by Professor N. Andry, whose book on the subject appeared in Paris in 1841; and its object, as its derivation from Greek implied, was the correction of deformities in children. As lateral curvature of the spine often developed in adolescence, however, it soon came to be used about treatments designed to correct deformities at that age, and eventually, at any age; and as orthopedists worked on bone and muscle – internal organs – they were regarded as, and called themselves, surgeons. And for some years they concentrated on finding ways to force, or cajole, the body back into its normal posture; inventing in the process a variety of types of brace, designed

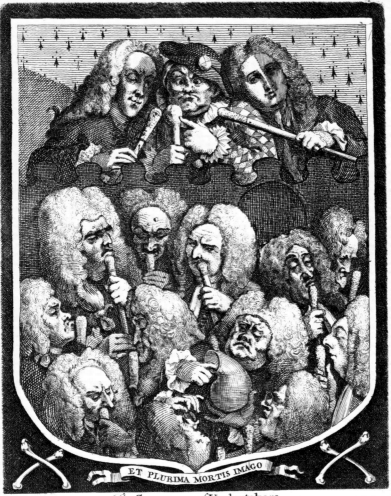

The Company of Undertakers

Beareth Sable, an Urinal *proper, between 12* Quack-Heads *of the second &* 12 Cane Heads *Or,* Consultant. *On a* Chief Nebulæ, *Ermine, One Compleat* Doctor *issuant, checkie sustaining in his*
Right Hand *a Baton of the second. On his* Dexter *&* sinister *sides two* Demi-Doctors, *issuant*
of the second, & two Cane Heads *issuant of the third; The first having One Eye* conchant, *to-*
wards the Dexter Side *of the Escocheon; the second* Faced *per pale proper & Gules, Guardent. ——*
With this Motto ———————— Et Plurima Mortis Imago.

Price Six pence

Publish'd by W. Hogarth. March the 3^d 1736

Hogarth's caricature coat of arms of medical practitioners; Sarah Mapp, a
celebrated bone-setter, appears in the top row. *Courtesy,* The Wellcome Trustees

to hold the spinal column straight. But to judge from the treatises on orthopedics in the period they did not consider simple backache to be their affair: it appears to have been left to the bone-setters.

The surgeons

Nevertheless it remained a standing reproach to surgeons, as they rose in the social world, that they could do so little for bad backs; and early in the 19th century Charles Bell, after experimenting in his own practice, claimed that he had found that some of them, at least, could be put right. There was no such thing as a dislocated back, he agreed, 'but a species of subluxation may certainly take place in the lumbar vertebrae'. This, he explained, was 'a dislocation of the articulating process, not of the bodies of the vertebrae, the invertebral substance being only a little irregularly stretched.'

Such derangements might be caused by wrestling, or fooling around, or by a weight falling on the shoulders when the body was bent forward; leading to the spinous 'processes' – the spine's knobbly outgrowths – getting entangled with each other. It was not easy to put them back because the body could not be twisted like an arm or a

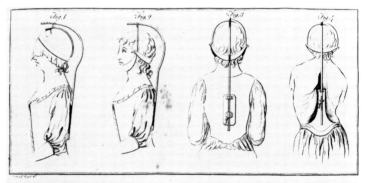

18th Century orthopaedic braces, designed to hold the spine straight. T. Sheldrake, *An Essay on the various Causes and Effects of the Distorted Spine*, 1783. *Courtesy, The Wellcome Trustees*

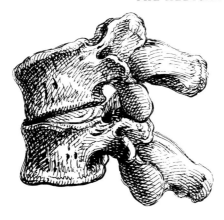

This drawing of dislocation of the articulating processes of the lumbar vertebrae was used to explain Charles Bell's theory in his handbook of surgery published in 1809. *Courtesy, The Wellcome Trustees*

leg; and even if it could have been, there would be a risk to the spinal cord. He admitted, however, that what appeared to be an accidental jolt sometimes did the trick. And sometimes the subluxation righted itself even when the surgeon could do nothing: 'in length of time, and by degrees', the spinous processes sorted themselves out, and the patient 'regained the erect posture'.

Bell's ideas were to be scornfully dismissed by the man who was establishing himself as the fashionable London surgeon of his time, Sir Astley Cooper, a Fellow of the Royal Society and surgeon to Guy's Hospital. In his *Treatise on Dislocations*, published in 1823, Cooper bluntly stated that derangements of the spine other than fracture, if they happened at all, were extremely rare; he personally had never seen a case. He had also, apparently, expressed himself even more forcibly on the subject (according to Bell, in terms 'revolting to good taste') in his lectures, which he had then circulated. Traditional ideas of treatment, Cooper insisted, were useless. The only way to deal with fractures was surgery, to fit the fractured vertebrae together again. The patient was bound to die if nothing was done, so that even if there were only one chance in a hundred, it was worth trying – 'notwithstanding any objections which some foolish persons may have urged against it'; anybody who said it ought not to be tried was 'a blockhead'.

The 'blockhead' – Bell, by this time surgeon to the Middlesex Hospital – replied the following year in his *Observations on Injuries of the Spine*. Cooper, he complained, had neither looked abroad, nor looked back in history; yet he delivered his 'hasty notions' with 'an air of commanding authority'. It was true that some of the most eminent medical writers had made mistakes; but that was no excuse for teaching students 'to despise the study of books, and to neglect all authority except that of the person addressing them, and all practice and example but that of the hospital to which chance had led them'. Cooper was right to deny the existence of spinal dislocations, other than fractures; but not to ignore the existence of subluxations, where the vertebrae were a little out of adjustment. In such cases there was no call for surgery. Manipulation could be tried; if it did not work, time might provide the cure. Cooper, Bell concluded, would have much to answer for 'in sending young men into practice with their heads full of dangerous notions about digging out the bones of the spine'.

Bell's warnings were ignored. Cooper became President of the Royal College of Surgeons, and was appointed surgeon to King George IV. For a time laminectomies, as the operations came to be called, were extensively practised. But the leaders of the next generation of fashionable surgeons, Robert Liston and Benjamin Brodie, came round to Bell's way of thinking; and though successes were claimed, no clear case was established of any patient recovering – as distinct from staying alive, but unable to walk. As for the mortality rate, although records were not kept, it must have been ugly – if only from infections caught during the operations. And this was still a time when there were no anesthetics to spare the patient agony on the operating table.

Searching for the causes

By the middle of the 19th century surgery for spinal disorders of any kind had been largely discredited. As has so commonly happened in the history of medicine when doctors were faced with a disorder which they did not understand, with no tradition of effective treatment to fall back on, they came to regard the whole field of orthopedics with distaste – in the United States, as well as in Europe. 'Its advancement has met with serious obstacles on the part of the profession', Louis Bauer, Professor of Clinical Anatomy and Surgery in New York, complained in one of his lectures, published in 1864.

All attempts at cultivating it had been 'frowned down as the pretences of quackery'.

Bauer himself had little to offer for backache, except rest and 'extension' – traction. He was mainly worried by the prevalence of curvature of the spine, which was confronting doctors with an intractable problem; 'few subjects of pathology have received more attention', he ruefully admitted, 'and in none have the combined efforts of scientific investigation been more barren of results'. So he had set out to see whether, even if he could not do anything for his patients, it might be possible to track down the causes, with a view to finding ways to prevent it – and perhaps backache, too. Both the immediate and the long term causes, he had found, were in dispute. Endless ideas had been put forward but none of them had proved acceptable. Some doctors assumed the weakness must be in the bones of the spine; others thought in terms of weakness in the spinal musculature. Bauer himself was inclined to believe that muscle strain was responsible, because he knew that the spinal vertebrae could be out of alignment without causing trouble. People with hunched shoulders, after all, were not necessarily incapacitated in any way, or in pain.

Whether an aching back was caused by some spinal derangement or by muscle strain might be of absorbing concern to doctors; for patients, the controversy was largely irrelevant, so long as the profession still had no acceptable treatment to offer – and the textbooks of the day reveal just how little to offer it had. *On Concussion of the Spine*, by John Eric Ericksen, Professor of Clinical Surgery at University College Hospital, London, appeared in 1875: it had over 300 pages on the pathology, diagnosis and prognosis of back disorders; in conclusion – almost as if added as an afterthought – a mere 12 pages sufficed for their treatment. Rest (the patient lying face downwards rather than on his back), along with 'diffusible stimulants, warm drinks, the repose of bed, and local application of fomentations', were all that Ericksen could confidently recommend.

'Cases that bone-setters cure'

In the circumstances, it was not surprising that patients began to look around for other ways to ease or remove their pain; and from time to time reports would appear about individuals whose doctors had been unable to do anything for them who had gone to a bone-setter for manipulation, and had been cured.

Manipulation had rarely been practised by physicians and surgeons. It had continued to be essentially a rural and working-class-urban form of treatment, makeshift, rude, and unprofessional. This was to be its undoing when, in the 1850s, the campaign to bring the teaching and practice of medicine under some control led to legislation to create the medical profession, very much as we know it today.

The process was not easy. The physicians regarded themselves as *the* medical profession, and would have preferred to retain their exclusivity. But by this time the surgeons, who had been careful to keep themselves distinct by continuing to style themselves 'Mr', had established themselves alongside the physicians in hospital hier-archies, and could not be excluded. Physicians and surgeons, too, because they were both hospital-trained, were united in their opposition to recognizing the humble apothecary as a doctor; he had usually learned his craft merely by apprenticeship. In all probability he would have been excluded, but for the fact that Members of Parliament were drawn from the landed gentry. As he looked after their families and their servants, he was in a good position to lobby successfully for recognition. This ought to have meant that the profession would continue to include men accustomed to manipulate as part of their job. But the price was that apothecaries must undertake the same medical training as physicians and surgeons; and as the training was given at teaching hospitals in the towns, the apprenticeship tradition was wiped out almost overnight. Hence-forth medical students, though they learned anatomy, physiology and pathology, and the theory of reducing fractures and dislo-cations, were given little if any opportunity to acquire the 'feel' of the bones and joints, ligaments and muscles of living people; and this made it difficult for general practitioners, as the former apothecaries came to be described, to practise manipulation.

The effects of this change were soon felt. Lecturing to his students in 1867 on injuries to bones and joints, the eminent surgeon James Paget told them he proposed to give them illustrations of the general principles he had laid down; and to secure their attention, he proposed to describe 'The Cases that Bone-Setters Cure'. Few of them, he warned, were likely to practise without having a bone-setter for a rival; 'and, if he can cure a case which you have failed to cure, his fortune may be made and yours marred'.

It was not that Paget had a high opinion of bone-setters. Their methods were crude – 'I believe that, in the large majority of cases, bone-setters treat injuries of joints, of whatever kind, with wrenching' – and their theories fallacious. It was impossible to measure the harm they did. But it was important for his students, he felt, to realize that the treatment sometimes did good: 'that by their practice of it, bone-setters live and are held in repute; and that their repute is, for the most part, founded on their occasionally curing a case which some good surgeon has failed to cure. For here, as in similar affairs, one success brings more renown than a hundred failures or mischiefs bring disgrace.'

It was consequently essential for doctors to recognize those cases where manipulation was indicated – apart from the reduction of dislocations, which was already part of a surgeon's training. They should know how to deal with slipped tendons and internal derangements of joints, or injured joints held stiff by involuntary muscular action, as sometimes happened with the cervical spine – the neck. 'From all this you may see that the cases that bone-setters cure are not a few. I think it very probable that those in which they do harm are numerous; but the lessons which you may learn from their practice are plain and useful.' Many more cases of injured joints than were commonly regarded as curable, he felt sure, could be successfully treated with 'wrenching, pulling and twisting'; and doctors should be able to deal with them. 'Learn, then', Paget concluded, 'to imitate what is good and avoid what is bad in the practice of bone-setters.'

'Doctors should learn to manipulate'

One doctor, Wharton Hood, took this advice – or perhaps had reached the same conclusion independently. In a series of articles in the *Lancet* in 1871, reprinted later in the year in a book, he described how he had accepted an offer from a well-known London bone-setter, Robert Hutton, to watch him at work; and as Hutton had since died, he no longer felt bound to preserve his secrets.

The theory on which Hutton and other bone-setters operated, Hood had found, was that they manipulated joints or vertebrae until a certain sound was heard, indicating to them (and to their patients) that a bone had popped back into place. This, Hood knew, was a fallacy. But there could be no question, he insisted, of Hutton's 'perfect good faith and honesty'; and there could also be no question that the method often worked – that pain was removed in this way

27

'by movements of flexion and extension, coupled with pressure on the painful spot'. It could even work for bone-setters when they set out to cure a hunchback in much the same way that Hippocrates had described. But it could be dangerous. The bone-setter

> every now and then cures conditions which the authorized practitioner had regarded with a sort of reverence because they were 'spinal'; and he every now and again kills a patient, because this reverence did not exist for his protection. If the profession generally would so study the diseases of the spinal cord as to rescue them from specialists, the first step would be taken towards rescuing the diseases of the vertebral column from quacks.

In a postscript to his earlier lecture, when it was reprinted in a collection of his work in 1875, Paget – by this time Sir James, and President of the Royal College of Surgeons – praised Hood 'who has so thoroughly learned the art, and practises it skilfully'; and added that there was another type of case, which he had not mentioned in his lecture, which bone-setters were said to cure, 'in which, after strains or other injuries of the spine, stiffness or aching long remain, and especially pain or tenderness over one spot at which, patients sometimes tell, a crack or slip was felt at the time of injury'. But he was still careful to insist that treatment by unqualified practitioners was not successful all or even most of the time, and that it could be dangerous. So he echoed his own and Hood's advice, that doctors themselves must learn how to manipulate.

Soon, this was to become a medical shibboleth. In a session on the subject at the annual meeting of the British Medical Association in 1882 Howard Marsh, a surgeon at St Bartholomew's, belittled the bone-setters – 'some are blacksmiths on the Cumberland hills, or shepherds in the sequestered valleys of Wales ... a very miscellaneous group, who resemble each other mainly in the negative point that they have never studied either anatomy, pathology or surgery', and warned that though some of them might use the techniques of orthodoxy, even anesthetics, they differed fundamentally from the profession in that 'diagnosis, properly so called, forms no part of their system'. As a result, they would miss vital diagnostic clues, and he claimed to have come across a number of cases where bone-setters had manipulated for what turned out to be bone tumors.

Nevertheless Marsh had to admit that in many cases, their methods worked; and in the discussion which followed, there was general agreement with his thesis. But nothing was done to implement Paget's proposal; for the simple reason that, given the structure of medical education, nothing *could* be done. So long as all medical students were trained in hospitals – and at that time, and for the best part of a century to come, virtually all their training was hospital-based – they had no opportunity to pick up the manipulator's craft. A few GPs might take the trouble to learn it, particularly if they practised in a working class area where there were industrial accidents, or at the other end of the social scale where men and women rode to hounds. But for the most part manipulation was left to the bone-setters: most of them part-timers (even Hutton was an upholsterer by trade); often blacksmiths and shepherds, as Marsh had described them, rarely known except in their locality.

ANDREW TAYLOR STILL: The father of osteopathy

In retrospect, it can be seen that the inability of the medical profession to make provision for manipulation was decisive. It would have been possible to set up a tributary organization, of the kind which promoted midwives from Mrs Gamp status to medical auxiliaries, enabling bone-setters to work within orthodoxy's network; but when this was not done the confrontation Paget had feared was inevitable. And as things turned out, it was much more serious than even he had foreseen. For by this time, the profession was faced with a more serious challenge than bone-setters, who had no organization and no prospect of forming one, could hope to provide: the introduction of the new manipulative schools, or cults – first osteopathy, and later chiropractic.

Andrew Taylor Still had been born in Virginia in 1828, the son of a farmer who was soon to migrate westward, as Abraham Lincoln's father had done earlier, in the familiar covered wagon. The medical schools of the mid-West at that time were designed in part to turn out the hob-nailed boot equivalent of Chairman Mao's barefoot doctors; youths were sent to them to pick up a smattering of medical knowledge designed for practice with the slaves on the parental farm, and in the neighbourhood. What Still learned as a student in one of them was presumably rudimentary. It sufficed, though, to qualify him to become an army doctor in the civil war – on the Union side, as he was an abolitionist; and after it ended he might have chosen to continue his career along orthodox lines, had not three of his children died in an epidemic of meningitis. Convinced there must be some better way to treat such diseases, he went back to the study of anatomy and physiology, coming to the conclusion that the secret of health lay in the liberation and purification of the blood stream. In the year 1874 he proclaimed that 'a disturbed artery marked the beginning to an hour and a minute when disease began to sow its seeds of destruction'. All diseases, he argued, were mere effects, the cause being the partial or complete failure of the blood properly to nourish the nervous system: 'interfere with the current of blood, and you steam down the river of life and land on the ocean of death'.

At the age of ten, Still recalled, suffering from a headache, he had made a 'pillow' by putting a blanket on a line slung between two trees; when he lay down with his neck on the blanket, he had been able to sleep, a method he had continued to use. The explanation, he surmised, was that it suspended the action of the occipital nerves at the back of the head, restoring the harmonious flow of the arterial blood to and through the veins. In the spinal cord, he now came to believe, lay the secret of stimulating that flow, with the help of manipulation and adjustment: a method which he proceeded to practise, to demonstrate, and to teach.

The teaching and the practice of medicine in the United States had not at that time come under the control of the hospital-based and city-based physicians and surgeons, as it had in Britain; and it might have been possible for a school of osteopathy, such as Still founded at Kirksville, Missouri, in 1892, to establish itself within the profession, or at least alongside it – much as schools of dentistry did. But there were difficulties. Although Still appears to have been a born manipulator, and a good teacher of manipulation, he could not describe how he did it, in writing – not, at least, in ways which would enable others to learn from the book, as distinct from watching him demonstrate.

Even more serious, the way that Still presented osteopathy meant that doctors could not regard him as an ally. It was in direct conflict with most of what they had been trained to believe. Diagnosis of the precise nature of a symptom, Still asserted, was of little importance, except in so far as it might be a guide to the part of the spine where the real trouble, a strain or a subluxation, would be found. If the spine was adjusted by manipulation, the blood flow would be

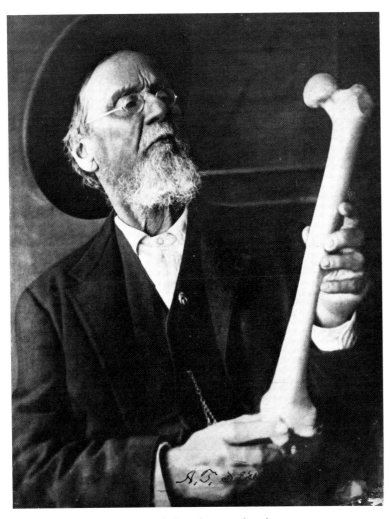

Andrew Taylor Still: The father of osteopathy who, as a young man, had served as an army doctor on the Union side.
Courtesy, British School of Osteopathy

restored to normal, and the symptom would disappear. 'All the remedies to human health exist in the human body', he insisted. 'They can be administered by adjusting the human body in such a manner that the remedies may naturally associate themselves together, hear the cries, and relieve the afflicted.'

To orthodoxy, this belief (and, doubtless, the high-flown language in which Still expressed himself), was lunacy. The idea that symptoms in other parts of the body could be caused by a 'spinal lesion' (as Still's concept came to be known) was rejected (even the notion of referred pain had slipped out of fashion) as implausible; and that adjustment could banish specific disorders like malaria, for which he advocated manipulation of the lower spine, or even dysentery, appeared grotesque.

Still did not himself employ the term 'lesion', but his followers did; not in its colloquial sense (so far as it can be said to have one) of a wound, but in its clinical sense of any kind of damage, or flaw, not necessarily specific. But the idea of 'the osteopathic lesion', which no pathologist had ever found, became a standing joke in the profession. And although Still did not claim that manipulation was a cure-all – his point was that orthodox medicine had no cures for the great majority of diseases; whereas the body, if suitably encouraged, might be roused to cure itself, a far from irrational point of view – the fact that osteopaths claimed manipulation could cure piles, or even get rid of tapeworms, was to doctors simply ludicrous.

D. D. PALMER: Founder of chiropractic

The medical profession was to be no more impressed by chiropractic, when it appeared 20 years after osteopathy. The founder, D. D. Palmer, claimed to have been unaware that another system of manipulation – osteopathy – existed; the story ran that he had developed the technique following a hunch which had prompted him to treat his office janitor's deafness by putting the heel of his hand to a lump in the man's neck, and giving a sharp thrust of the kind Hippocrates had described. The school of spinal manipulation which grew up around Palmer tended to concentrate on the neck; and, following his example, to use a more abrupt manipulative technique. His chiropractic theory, too, put less emphasis on the role of the blood, and more on the belief that spinal subluxations or displacements impinged on the nerves issuing from the spinal column. But both schools shared the view that health is dependent upon spinal adjustment, and that illness of any kind can best be treated by correcting maladjustments manipulatively. Both, inevitably, were put under the medical profession's interdict.

The divergence between their point of view and orthodoxy's was not quite so fundamental as it seemed. A. H. Tubby, for example, a London surgeon and a paragon of medical orthodoxy, was prepared in his textbook, first published in 1890, to accept the proposition that some physical disorders (as well as referred pain) might originate in the spine; he cited the example of a link which had been found between herpes (shingles) and vertebral decay, which had prompted the suggestion that cases of shingles might be the consequence of a lesion in the spinal column. In retrospect, too, it seems likely that even if the manipulators could not do what they boasted they could do, their methods must have been at least as effective as most of the remedies then in everyday use, and a great deal safer. ('Percy Driscoll had had children round his hearthstone', as Mark Twain sombrely put it in *Pudd'nhead Wilson* in 1894; 'but they had been attacked in detail by measles, croup and scarlet fever, and this had given the doctor a chance with his antediluvian methods, and the cradles were empty'.) At the time, though, osteopathy and chiropractic could only appear as a threat to doctors' faith, as well as to their livelihood; and, in their eyes, a menace to patients who put themselves at the mercy of such charlatans. Had not Pasteur recently disclosed the way that disease-producing germs, hitherto undiscovered, were the cause of infectious diseases? Had not Koch just isolated the bacillus which caused tuberculosis? Was it seriously to be claimed that these invaders could be routed by an ignorant manipulator, fumbling at the victim's spine?

HERBERT BARKER: 'An impertinent one-man campaign'

At the turn of the century, and indeed on up to the second world war, the medical profession in the United States was not yet well-organized enough to exercise full control over its own members, let alone breakaway groups. But in Britain the General Medical Council was legally entitled to investigate, arraign, put on trial, and excommunicate any doctor by erasing his name from the Medical Register, if in its members' opinion he had shown himself unworthy to practise medicine: and one of the GMC's rules was that doctors must not refer patients to, or work in conjunction with, any medically unqualified practitioner, other than one who was licensed as an auxiliary, such as a qualified nurse. The design was to protect the patient from lazy or unscrupulous doctors, and to keep him out of the clutches of quacks. But as Paget had warned, if there were some

33

form of treatment which doctors could not or would not provide, patients would be tempted to go to a quack anyway; and a quack emerged, in Herbert Barker, who came quite close to confounding the profession single-handed.

His career is worth examining in some detail, for its revelation of a fundamental weakness of the profession; its inability to adapt itself to the fact that there may be some forms of treatment which owe their success more to some indefinable quality in the practitioner, than to the method he uses.

As a youth in the 1880s, following a serious illness, Barker was prescribed an open air life in Canada; and on the ship crossing the Atlantic he found himself, without premeditation, and guided by instinct, 'reducing' – re-positioning – a fellow passenger's dislocated elbow. It happened that Barker had a cousin, John Atkinson, who had trained under Robert Hutton as a bone-setter, and had gone on to acquire a fashionable London practice, his clients including the musician Paderewski and the C. in C. of the British Army, the Duke of Cambridge. On his return from Canada, Barker apprenticed himself to his cousin; then set up for himself for some years in Manchester; and in 1906 came back to practise in London.

Barker was not primarily a manipulator of the spine. He had been making his living, and his reputation, chiefly from his ability to straighten out twisted knees, ankles and other joints of the kind footballers commonly suffered from; and by restoring arches to children's flat feet. But one of the commonest disorders at that time – particularly in adolescence, to judge from contemporary medical writings – was scoliosis: curvature of the spine to one side or the other. And as scoliosis was notoriously a vexing problem to doctors, Barker had plenty of practice manipulating spines.

The method which he followed with joints which had come out of their correct alignment was the age-old one by which bone-setters reduced dislocations and fractures: freeing the displaced surfaces of the joint, and then maneuvering them around until they fell into place – sometimes with a characteristic sound which was believed to indicate that they *were* in place, like the 'pop' some people like to make cracking their finger joints. First, he had to clear the way for his operation by breaking down the 'adhesions' – the temporary fencing, as it were, which the body put up around an injured or dislocated joint to protect it in its new position. It was to this craft, or knack, Hood thought – and Paget agreed – that bone-setters largely owed their success; and Barker's particular skill appears to have lain in estimating precisely the degree of force to use, and where to apply it, in order to make the joint surfaces mobile. He could then restore the proper alignment. It could be painful, but it was usually quick, and often permanent, except with those cases of people, common enough, who suffered from recurrent dislocations for no obvious reason.

Actions rather than words

With backs, Barker worked on the same principle, though for obvious reasons they required a rather different technique. He found it hard to describe precisely what he did, but he was always willing to demonstrate to doctors, and one of them was later to describe in the *Lancet* what he had witnessed. The patient had been suffering from lower back pains which had left her barely able to walk; and she had not responded to medical treatment. Brought to Barker, she was put lying prone on a couch, and he proceeded to go through two motions.

> With one hand on the sacrum, the other under the left shoulder, the operator forcibly extended and rotated the trunk a few times in rapid succession while keeping the pelvis immobile on the couch. The second movement was done while the patient was prone as before. One hand being on the sacrum keeping the trunk on the couch, the other hand was applied below both knees in such a way as to over-extend the hip and lumbo-sacral joints. Both movements required great muscular effort, and during each, sounds as of giving-way of adhesions were clearly heard.

The patient was immediately relieved, the doctor reported, and after a repeat performance a week later had 'remained quite well since'.

Barker was an operator, not a theorist. He was convinced that his methods, for whatever reason, gave good results, and he knew that he was doing what doctors could not, or at any rate did not, attempt to do; but as he could not explain his technique in print, he must persuade them to come and see for themselves. He had made contacts with the press in Manchester, and soon after he came down to London he persuaded the *Daily Express* to sponsor a trial with eight patients who had been told by their doctors that nothing could be done for them: he successfully cured seven of them, and the eighth greatly benefited. When these results were ignored, Barker wrote to

35

a number of eminent medical men begging them to investigate; his letters, too, were ignored. The only reaction he obtained was hostile comment in the *British Medical Journal*. But this, to the editor's surprise, brought in a shoal of correspondence from (as a further editorial admitted) 'archdeacons, priests, professors of engineering, heroes of the football field, and members of fashionable ladies' clubs' – Barker's grateful patients.

What followed may have been coincidental, but in view of later developments was more probably linked to Barker's impertinent one-man campaign. In 1908, the General Medical Council passed a resolution calling on the Government to investigate 'the evil effects produced by the unrestricted practice of medicine and surgery by unqualified persons'. The Government, however, obliged only half-heartedly, by circularizing Medical Officers of Health for their opinions; and when the report of their views was published in 1910, though it confirmed there were many 'illiterate and unlearned' bone-setters, it had to admit that in some districts they enjoyed 'a large amount of public confidence'. In the North of England the Friendly Society of which almost all miners were members actually accepted disability certificates from bone-setters as the equivalent of certificates from doctors. Asquith's Government in that year had more important matters to worry about; it was able to extricate itself from the need to take any action by arguing that bone-setting was not a public health problem.

The 'undeveloped land' of medicine

That autumn, there appeared what to Barker and his supporters was the first sign of a change of heart in the profession. The *British Medical Journal* carried an article by Alexander Bryce, who had been studying osteopathy in America, in which he described the objectives of 'mechano-therapy', as he called it. Diagnosis, he explained, was concerned not with the symptoms of a disorder, but with a spinal lesion; 'a structural change affecting function', such as a sub-luxation, thickened ligaments, or contracted muscles – and treatment was by manipulation. 'I do not hesitate to plead for the admission of the new form of scientific bone-setting among the recognized forms of treatment', he concluded: 'if we deny the possibility of the existence of so-called subluxations – as is the custom with medical men – we lay ourselves open to the charge of perpetuating the presence of such irregular practitioners in our midst'.

It was surprising enough that the editor of the *B.M.J.* should have accepted an article preaching such heresy; but even more astonishing, in view of his past attitude, was the accompanying editorial on the 'undeveloped land' of medicine, insisting that medicine 'to be truly rational, must refuse to be bound within the trammels of any system; in a scientific sense it must be non-sectarian', and going on to urge that therapies like 'the higher bone-setting' should not be dismissed with a foolish contempt, but should be studied, and 'the secret of whatever good there may be in them should be discovered'.

As Barker was to recall in his autobiography, the *B.M.J.*'s words sounded to him like the crackling noise which proclaimed the break-up of the ice packs, 'when the waters of a great river feel the breath of spring'. But he very soon found that he was not to be a beneficiary of the thaw. A few weeks later, when he was sued by a youth who had come for treatment with a tuberculous leg, which had later been amputated, the *B.M.J.* was not disposed to be sympathetic.

Again, it may have been coincidence that the case was brought at a time when Barker's persistent campaigning for recognition was causing so much irritation in the profession. If the youth's family had been egged on to bring the case, though, it proved a weak choice. Barker was able to show that he had not manipulated the knee; he had merely examined it. He had, however, sent the boy for palliative heat treatment, rather than referring him back to his doctor; this, coupled with the fact that on his own admission he made a wretched show in the witness box, and that Mr Justice Darling summed up strongly against him, led the jury to find for the plaintiff; and though the damages were derisory, Darling awarded the full costs of the case against Barker. As Sir Edward Clarke had led for the plaintiff and Sir Edward Carson for the defence, the expense was formidable. The verdict, too, meant that it would always be possible for Barker's critics to remind their readers that he had been convicted of negligence; an advantage which some of them were duly to exploit.

Official harassment

Had the medical Establishment been content to ignore Barker, at this point, he might well have decided to lie low, in future, and not risk another humiliation. But – and this time it can hardly have been coincidence – the General Medical Council could not resist intervening to harass him still further. As he was not on the Register, they could not touch him; but he was assisted by F. W. Axham, a doctor who had been so impressed by Barker's methods that he had offered his services as an anesthetist, though realizing the risk he ran. He had been working in this capacity for six years without any action being taken against him; but he had appeared as a key witness in Barker's defence, and this could not be condoned. Axham was charged with associating with an unregistered person; and when he refused to give an assurance that the association would cease, his name was erased from the Register. It was also removed from the membership roll of the Royal College of Physicians in Edinburgh, and of the Royal College of Surgeons in London.

By its action, so palpably spiteful, the GMC succeeded only in turning press and public over to Barker's side. W. T. Stead, the most experienced campaigning editor in Fleet Street, had already come out on his side; now, Barker's and Axham's case was to be enthusiastically endorsed in a number of the popular dailies, in the still influential magazine *Truth*, and even in *The Times*, which in 1912 carried an article 'What is a Quack?', making the point that as it 'would be utterly ridiculous to pretend to doubt that Mr Barker has effected perfect cures where regular surgeons have failed', he should not be thus described, because the term was intended to carry a moral stigma.

It was time, Sir Rickman Godlee, President of the Royal College of Surgeons, decided, to exert his authority; and he chose to criticize the bone-setters not for their manipulative method, but for their fallacious diagnostic claims. If the writer of *The Times'* article went to a bone-setter with a strained back, Godlee replied, if he were told that vertebrae were dislocated, and if he gained relief from the treatment, he would naturally assume that the explanation of his cure was correct; 'some knowledge of pathology is required to appreciate the impossibility of the diagnosis, or the ignorant boasting of the bone-setter who, in spite of his successes, is justly dubbed a quack'. Godlee was careful not to name Barker; but it was obviously Barker to whom he was referring, and Barker seized the opportunity to make him look ridiculous by quoting orthodox authorities more eminent in the field than Godlee himself in refutation. Professor John Ericksen, Barker was able to show, had accepted that the spine could be partially dislocated; 'whilst one of the highest and most modern authorities', Rosswell Park, had asserted that 'a limited proportion of serious injuries to the spine consists of dislocation of some of its component parts'. Barker was even able to slide in some self-promotion. He had just treated a doctor's wife whose painful spinal complaint had for years resisted the attentions of the best surgeons in London; 'it has responded to manipulative treatment so well that the patient has made a complete recovery'.

Powerful champions

The controversy spluttered on until the outbreak of the first world war, in which Barker gave free treatment to men in the ranks with such impressive results that in 1916 a group of his patients – they included Lord William Cecil, Admiral Kerr, Major General Sir William Hamilton and H. G. Wells – supported by 50 MPs, petitioned the War Office to utilize his services. The War Office replied that King's Regulations would not permit such an appointment. After the war ended, Barker's supporters tried another tack: no less than 300 past and present MPs, including the Lord Chancellor and 13 Privy Councillors, petitioned the Archbishop of Canterbury to use the power which he still possessed, under the Act setting up the medical profession, to grant Barker an honorary medical degree. The Archbishop declined, but urged that some other way should be found to mark appreciation of Barker's 'eminent services to sufferers'. Soon after, a way was found: Barker was knighted.

Barker's career makes a dramatic story in its own right; but in the context of the history of the search for understanding of the human back, it is chiefly significant for its revelation of the vindictive obstructiveness of the medical profession when confronted with an outsider who can treat patients successfully where its recommended orthodox methods have failed.

Nobody has since come near to repeating Barker's phenomenal success, but there are today scores of competent practitioners of manipulation who are not qualified doctors, and the arguments used against them are still precisely the same as those which were used against him – with one exception. Barker knew little of osteopathy or chiropractic, neither of which had yet established itself outside the United States. He remained a bone-setter, manipulating in order to reduce dislocations or maladjustments – not with a view to curing other forms of disease. It could not therefore be said of him, as it was about osteopaths and chiropractors, that their own absurdly inflated pretensions put them out of court. But all the other stock criticisms of osteopaths and chiropractors were made of him – most of them by Sir William Watson Cheyne in the House of Commons in 1917, when he was defending the army's decision not to take in Barker.

Barker by this time had too many influential backers for a frontal assault to be wise; so Cheyne patronizingly conceded his 'good work' and settled for the thin-end-of-the-wedge line; if Barker were admitted, how could other bone-setters be excluded? Bone-setters had no formal training in diagnosis: therefore they might easily miss some vital clue, and use manipulation on a tubercular bone, with disastrous results. And were they really all that successful? Even where they succeeded, the results were apt to be temporary. In any case, there was nothing which the bone-setter could do which a good orthopedic surgeon could not do just as well. And if a bone-setter really had talent, why should he not become a medical student?

In Barker's case, these arguments were hollow. Although he had had no formal training, his apprenticeship had given him experience which, allied to natural skill, had put him far ahead of the orthopedic surgeons of his time. That he had had no training in diagnosis, and might therefore manipulate when what the patient was suffering from was a tuberculous bone, was superficially a more convincing line – especially after the court case. Barker, however, claimed not merely that he could detect such cases, but that sometimes manipulation was actually effective – certainly much more likely to be effective, he insisted, than the orthodox method of immobilization, which made matters worse. But the criticism was in any event misdirected. The overwhelming majority of Barker's patients, even after he became famous, came to him after they had been seen, investigated and treated – or turned away – by doctors. If they had TB, or cancer, or any other such disease, it was their doctors who had missed it, first. And in Barker's case, it is scarcely possible that he made any really serious diagnostic error. With so much publicity surrounding his work, and so many enemies ready to pounce, it could not have been hushed up.

That he had some failures, Barker himself admitted; and in some cases he would not even attempt treatment. But there is one indication that the failure rate must have been low. In 1917 an anonymous letter in the *Sunday Times* called on patients of Barker who felt dissatisfied to specify their complaints by writing to the Royal Society of Medicine. The invitation apparently brought in a flood of letters testifying to Barker's skill, but nothing which could be used against him.

Nor is there anything that suggests that Barker's cures were

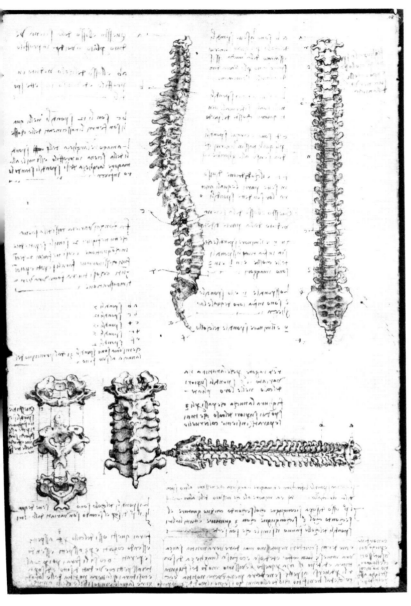

Leonardo da Vinci's drawing of the spine; the first to show the articulated human vertebral column with the vertebrae correctly numbered in each part.
Reproduced by gracious permission of Her Majesty The Queen

temporary. On the contrary, he could produce a mass of testimony that they were lasting; and on the only publicized occasion when it was challenged – by Lord Knutsford in 1917 with the assertion that a man whom Barker claimed to have cured of a dislocated spine was as crippled as before within two months – Barker was able to reply that on the contrary, so effective had his treatment been that the man had been able to rejoin the forces, and was actually at the Front.

As for the argument that orthopedic surgeons could do what Barker did as well or better, a surgeon who had himself been successfully treated by Barker pointed out that the manipulation described in medical textbooks was 'like snakes in Ireland: it doesn't exist, and never has existed'. He had seen orthopedic surgeons practising manipulation, and had tried it himself; but it was utterly different from Barker's techniques.

Closing of the ranks

The final argument – that if a bone-setter wanted to be treated as a doctor, he should qualify – was to be brought up by the Secretary to the General Medical Council at the time when the idea of a Lambeth Degree (one awarded by the Archbishop of Canterbury under powers that had survived since the middle ages) was being canvassed; 'it was open to Mr Barker, or anyone, to seek a degree in the ordinary way, and be registered'. When Oxford or Cambridge awarded an honorary degree in music, Bernard Shaw replied, 'we have not found uppish village organists informing the *Daily Telegraph* that "it is open to Mr Brahms, or any one else, to seek a degree in the ordinary way", by doing exercises in obsolete counterpoint'. All professions, Shaw had asserted in *The Doctor's Dilemma* – written before Barker became famous, otherwise he would surely have featured in it, in some role – are conspiracies against the laity; and there could hardly have been a better illustration than the General Medical Council which, he now observed, was exhibiting every constitutional vice a profession could have. It was not doctors: it was their profession – or, rather, their professional Establishment: the interlocking groups who ran the GMC and the Colleges and advised Governments, whose members often thought and acted differently in their Establishment capacity than as individuals – which fought Barker, and what he stood for. Some of the most eminent medical men of his time supported him: Walter Whitehead, a former President of the BMA, had offered to give evidence for him at his trial;

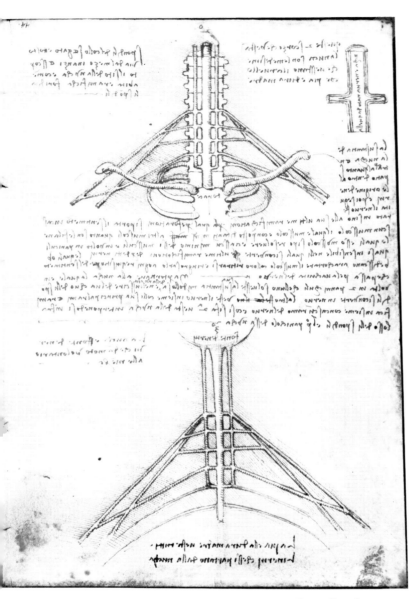

Leonardo's drawing (top) shows a spinal cord sawn in half revealing the nerves running from the brain above down the spinal cord, then spreading out on either side to form the brachial plexus. (Below) The base of the brain, the spinal cord and brachial plexus removed from the bones and membranes that enclosed them. Leonardo believed, wrongly, that the spinal cord was made up of one central and two lateral channels. *Reproduced by gracious permission of Her Majesty The Queen*

and among those who advised the Prime Minister in favour of his knighthood were the Royal Surgeon, Sir Alfred Fripp, and Sir William Arbuthnot Lane. Whatever surgeons of that standing might personally think, though, in their capacity as pillars of the medical Establishment they felt they had to continue to support it, in case the whole edifice might crumble under the onslaught of this unexpected Samson in their midst. And whatever their personal inclinations, as members of the GMC they were prepared to continue to thwart him, and to defy public opinion.

When Barker was knighted Axham had retired. He was by this time in his eighties; the general assumption was that as a conciliatory gesture his name would be restored to the Medical Register, and to the rolls of the Royal Colleges of which he had been a member. This was the course publicly urged by Lord Dawson of Penn, King George V's physician. The Royal College of Physicians in Edinburgh took it, excusing itself by pointing out that Axham had ceased to practise. The Royal College of Surgeons in London, and the General Medical Council, rejected the plea. A few weeks later, Axham died.

It could not even be argued that the members of the General Medical Council were being consistent: that they were being cruel to an individual only to protect the public from unqualified practitioners, as their rules laid down. They had deprived themselves of that excuse, because they had not dared to erase from the Register the name of Axham's successor as Barker's anesthetist. They did not have to account for this decision; but the reason was obvious. Had they taken any such action the outcry would have been so vehement, and the support for retaliatory action so powerful, that legislation would almost certainly have been brought in to curtail the GMC's power. Its members were making their public stand on an issue of principle; privately, they were guided by the instinct of professional self-preservation.

THE BONE-SETTERS' LEGACY

The bone-setter tradition was to leave one other legacy, of a different kind: an infiltration into orthodoxy which was profoundly to change attitudes to orthopedics.

The Thomases

In many parts of Britain, bone-setting had been passed on for

generations from father to son; and one such family were the
Thomases of Anglesey in North Wales. Even before the 1858 Act
which set up the medical profession, Evan Thomas had decided that
it would be wise for his sons, if they wanted to practise, to qualify as
doctors; and Hugh Owen Thomas duly did, setting up in practice in
Liverpool. He treated patients with a blend of bone-setting and
orthodox conservative treatment, using the techniques his father had
used, but cautiously, and employing orthopedic aids like plaster casts
– introduced in the 1870s as a way to keep the body or neck in place
after traction. He was not, like Barker, a keen manipulator; he
believed in letting the body alone, to do its own repair work.

His practice soon became extensive: treating children with
disorders of the spine or limbs, often resulting from malnutrition,
and dockers with sprains or fractures. Perhaps because he worked in
Liverpool, his fame spread across the Atlantic, leading to visits from
American orthopedic surgeons – who were just as uncertain as their
English counterparts as to how to treat many of their patients. One of
them, Dr John Ridlon of Chicago, was fascinated to watch him at
work reducing dislocations – for traditionally, bone-setters could
perform that operation with the apparent facility of a chef breaking
eggs into a mixing bowl. But there was something which Thomas felt
keenly, Ridlon found: that the physicians and surgeons 'looked
down upon him as a bone-setter; that he was ostracized pro-
fessionally'. And when his nephew Robert Jones came up to
Liverpool after qualifying, to work as his assistant, he found that
Thomas had 'preached as one in the wilderness'; his work had been
either ignored or discountenanced.

The resistance to the adoption of the bone-setters' methods, then,
was not simply a matter of professional resentment of outsiders. It
was also derived from snobbery (doctors, as Shaw described in the
preface to *The Doctor's Dilemma*, were moving up in the world
socially, and did not care to be identified with so working class a
method); and from professional jealousy – because Thomas was
making a success of a method they could only imitate, and that not
satisfactorily. For as Thomas had written, soon after he began to
practise, 'my father and I are the practitioners of an art that does not
belong to the exact sciences'. Even with the best application of that
art, he admitted, things often went wrong, 'and again many times a
course of treatment not to be justified by either reason or experience
succeeds.'

The physicians and surgeons might dismiss him: what the people of Liverpool felt about Thomas was to be shown when he died in 1891. There could be no more eloquent testimony – a local reporter wrote, describing the funeral –

> to the worth of a man's character than the tears of the poor among whom he lived. The toilers of our docks and warehouses are no sensitive beings, and the daily struggle of their lives is too earnest to admit of much display of sentiment. To see thousands of these, then, men as well as women, as anyone might have done in Liverpool last Saturday, stirred to their very depths by an emotion that found expression in passionate sobs and tears, as they lined the streets or pressed forward to look into the open grave, proves that its silent occupant had won its way to their hearts . . .

Yet Hugh Owen Thomas would have been forgotten, in all probability, had it not been for his apprentice, Robert Jones, who took over his practice.

Sir Robert Jones

Jones was one generation and one social step removed from the bone-setter stigma; and with his talent and energy he was able to break out of general practice into consultant posts, and up into the medical Establishment. And in doing so, he managed to bring respectability to orthopedic surgery. Partly because orthopedics offered so little in the way of effective measures to treat patients but also, probably, because of a deep-laid revulsion about 'cripples', it had remained low in the hierarchy of medical specialties. Almost single-handed, Jones was to instil active enthusiasm for it. He had the advantage, too, of x-rays; he was among the first to import a machine to Britain – though as it happened, he was also one of the first to express dissatisfaction with the way in which radiography came to be used by colleagues and students as a substitute for, rather than as a way of confirming, a clinical diagnosis. Soon, by a combination of his own skill, the techniques he had learned from Thomas, and the latest orthopedic gadgetry, he was able not merely to effect remarkable cures but also to convince his colleagues that he was pursuing an orthodox and scientific course.

It was to no purpose, even though Jones himself added to his stature during the war. Unlike Barker, he could be employed by the army, using his talents to the full; and when the war ended, he was able to return to devote his full energies to the setting up of the first fully-fledged orthopedic department in a London teaching hospital, and later a network of orthopedic centres throughout Britain. And it is hard to overestimate Jones's importance in the campaign which followed against spinal diseases. Thirty years earlier he had emphasized the importance of improving social conditions: better housing, recreation grounds, fresh air, purer food, safer milk – all these, he had insisted, were required to bring about the day 'when we poor physicians and surgeons, many of us at least, may be relegated to the ranks of the unemployed'; and in the 1920s he continually and successfully strove for the eradication of TB and rickets by such measures as eliminating bovine TB which was often transmitted to children through drinking cows' milk. As a result there was a marked improvement in children's bones, including their vertebrae; and soon, far fewer cases of deformity.

But remarkable though his achievement was, it had the paradoxical effect of blocking the introduction of manipulative techniques of the kind Barker and osteopaths used. Jones himself was a manipulator – 'of astounding ability', according to the celebrated Italian surgeon Professor Putti; but his manipulation appears to have been chiefly concerned with limbs, rather than with spines, and he used it mainly to break down adhesions and correct deformities. Orthopedists tended to use him as their model, rather than Barker or the osteopaths. Jones and Barker might have lived on different planets. In a book which was presented to Jones on his birthday in 1928, one of the 24 articles by the distinguished contemporaries who contributed to it was on spinal curvature, another on the association of certain intestinal conditions with arthritis, and two on spinal disorders in infancy; but there was no article on backache, or its treatment.

Victory for the manipulators

One last attempt was to be made to bring the orthopedists and the manipulators together. Barker had retired; but in 1936 he was invited by the authorities at St Thomas's Hospital in London to give a demonstration of his technique on 18 patients who had not benefited from orthodox treatment, presenting him with a variety of the kinds of joint disorder in whose treatment he had made his reputation. Publication of the results was delayed until the following year, to give the scrutineers the opportunity to check on how lasting the improvement, if any, would be. According to the report in the *Lancet*, Barker had been allowed some latitude in his choice of suitable patients to treat; but it was conceded that he had not selected only the easier cases. Yet after the follow-up, ten of them were pronounced cured; five were improved; and there were only three failures.

The Times led its Home News section the next day with a summary of the *Lancet*'s report, and in a leading article observed that the need for further demonstration was obvious. If Barker's contentions were confirmed, 'then steps ought to be taken at once to make such teaching as widely available as possible not only to British surgeons but to surgeons in all parts of the world'. It would be a calamity, *The Times* felt, to deprive sufferers of such help. But happily, precedent was on the side of wisdom; 'medicine and surgery are the beneficiaries of a host of extra-mural workers, every one of whom in his day had to fight the battle for recognition'. Such battles might be necessary for purposes of testing, 'but when they have been won there is no longer excuse for opposition or even for inaction'.

It was a tactful way of reminding the medical Establishment both how obscurantist, and how wrong, it had been in the past, and also how quickly all would be forgotten and forgiven if it now saw the light. But it underestimated the strength of the opposition, and of inertia. St Thomas's continued to provide Barker with facilities, in particular to make films of his technique – one of the problems still being that it was so difficult for him or anybody else to describe it in print in meaningful terms. In the summer of 1939 *The Times* again led its Home News one day with a column on the subject, describing how he had been filmed while at work on various parts of the body, including the lower spine, and recalling some of the distinguished men who had testified to his skill, including the Duke of Kent, Earl Beatty, John Galsworthy, Lord Hawke, and Georges Carpentier the heavy-weight boxer. 'There will be universal satisfaction', an editorial claimed,

> that the methods of manipulative surgery introduced and practised by Sir Herbert Barker have now been placed upon permanent record in a form suitable for the training of students . . . thanks to these films all further generations will be able to avail themselves of a body of knowledge and experience of which so many in this present generation are the beneficiaries.

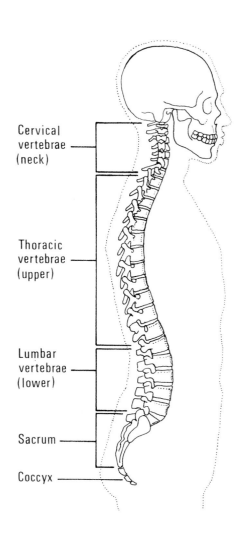

Cervical
vertebrae
(neck)

Thoracic
vertebrae
(upper)

Lumbar
vertebrae
(lower)

Sacrum

Coccyx

The spinal column

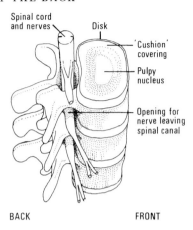

Spinal cord and nerves

Disk

'Cushion' covering

Pulpy nucleus

Opening for nerve leaving spinal canal

BACK   FRONT

A detailed section of the lumbar spine.

'My labours have not been in vain', Barker delightedly told *The Times*. 'The battle for manipulative surgery is won.' But battles of a more serious nature were imminent; a few weeks later, Hitler's forces moved into Poland. When Britain declared war normal teaching hospital routine was shelved, at St Thomas's as elsewhere in London, in the expectation that the beds would be required for the victims of the blitz which would inevitably follow – as, nearly a year later, it did. During the war, surgery for backache came back into fashion again; and after it, the rise of the 'wonder drugs', in particular cortisone and its steroid derivatives, gave the impression for a time that the controversy over manipulation was of no more than historical interest. And it is at this point that it becomes simpler to separate out the strands, and to look at the options through the eyes of a present day patient, wondering what course to take.

The Options

1 Orthodoxy's Ways

To go back, then, to where we started. Lying in bed, with nothing stronger than aspirin prescribed to ease your pain, you may well begin to wonder why your doctor has not recommended surgery. It is very possible, for example, that he has told you your trouble is, or may be, a 'slipped disk'. Whatever happened to the operations that, not many years ago, were the standard form of treatment? If it really is simply a displaced disk which is causing the trouble – and with all the diagnostic gadgetry available, this should surely be easy to determine – why can't an operation be arranged to end the pain once and for all?

The answer, again, lies in history; not in the contest between Bell and Astley Cooper, though that can now be seen to have presented a salutary early warning, but in what has been happening during the last 50 years.

SURGICAL TREATMENT

Surgeons had never entirely lost hope of finding a way to cure backache; but when eventually they did find it, the operation was not at all of the kind which Cooper and his disciples had sought to perfect. Medical orthodoxy increasingly frowned on vague diagnosis; the search for specific organic causes of pain was intensified; and in the 1920s the explanation 'focal sepsis' began to enjoy a vogue. Ironically, it was almost a carbon copy of Cutler Walpole's 'nuciform sac' theory in Shaw's play, *The Doctor's Dilemma*, attributing all illness to foci of infection. They might be found anywhere in the body; and anywhere they were found, they were excised, the notion being that ills and aches of many kinds, including backache, were the result of the infection emanating from them. As many people had rotten teeth and inflamed tonsils, these were considered to be the commonest foci: 'one almost never saw an arthritic who had not lost his teeth and his tonsils', Weiss and English were later to recall in their medical textbook.

It was perhaps the cruellest and craziest – for there was never any convincing evidence for the theory – surgical orgy of all time. Even if a surgeon was not convinced that the theory was sound, he might still feel compelled to send his patients to be checked for focal sepsis, and if it were found, to recommend an operation. In his book *Backache*, published in 1931, the vastly experienced Emeritus Professor of Medicine at Johns Hopkins, L. F. Barker, was prepared to commit himself only to the proposition that focal infections were 'believed to be' a cause of back pain; yet though he knew of cases where no foci had been found, and also of cases where they had been found but where the patient had recovered without their being removed, he nevertheless felt compelled to recommend that all foci of infection 'should be eradicated as early as possible', to be on the safe side. And many patients, aware that medical science had no alternative treatment to offer, actually welcomed the operation, under the not uncommon delusion that the more far-fetched the diagnosis, and the more savage the treatment, the greater must surely be the likelihood of a cure.

Operations for focal sepsis went out of fashion painfully slowly; but patients with backache were rescued by the discovery that another, more specific operation could be employed, based on the belief that one of the chief causes might be a fault in one of the intervertebral disks.

The ruptured disk

The existence of intervertebral disks, or discs – biscuit-shaped spinal shock-absorbers with a tough, though springy, outer cover of cartilage containing a pulpy, gelatinous substance – had been known for centuries, but they had not been suspected of being trouble-makers until Edgar F. Cyriax, a London doctor with osteopathic leanings, suggested in 1919 that what he described as 'disc-luxations' might cause backache; his reasoning being that its symptoms sometimes resembled those caused in other joints by displaced fragments of cartilage. Later, the German pathologist George Schmorl reported that he had occasionally found leakage of the pulp through the disk's cover in post mortems; and in 1934 the *New England Journal of Medicine* carried an account by two Boston surgeons, W. J. Mixter and J. S. Barr, describing how they had encountered a number of cases which had originally been diagnosed as tumors, but which had turned out to be ruptured disks.

In retrospect Mixter and Barr's paper has come to be regarded as heralding a new era; but it took some time for its significance to sink in, perhaps because it could be construed as giving aid and comfort to the osteopaths and chiropractors. They had always claimed that backache was caused by a spinal lesion: now, here was the demonstration that a spinal lesion could indeed be the cause. The osteopaths and chiropractors, however, were a little chary of claiming credit: partly because they had had in mind a rather different kind of lesion – displacement or subluxation of the vertebrae – and partly because the notion of a ruptured disk being responsible for back pain was promptly challenged. 'As this subject is still *sub judice*', Macdonald and Wilson cautiously commented in their 1935 survey of osteopathy, 'we shall content ourselves with mentioning it in passing'.

Gradually, however, orthopedic surgeons and neurosurgeons came to realize that if ruptured disks could be held responsible for back pain, a whole new prospect lay open to them, awaiting their scalpels. Laminectomy had long been out of favour; here was the chance to try an alternative form of spinal operation – 'diskectomy'. The disk operation, too, had a distinct advantage over its predecessor. So far as was known the disk's only function was to act as a shock absorber, so that it could be tinkered with, or scooped out, without affecting other organs – except the vertebrae above and below; and they could be operated upon and if necessary fused, or stapled, together, to prevent jarring that would otherwise occur.

The second world war provided a perfect opportunity for experiment. A very common form of casualty were back injuries caused when tanks or trucks ran into pot holes, or were blown up by mines. It was relatively simple to open up the patient's back, to check whether a disk had ruptured; if so, it could be removed; if not, no harm was done – and no expense incurred by the patient. A few months after the war ended two British surgeons, B. H. Burns and R. H. Young, described in the *Lancet* how they had operated upon 140 patients who had been found to have disk lesions, and who had not responded to rest or lumbar corsets within three weeks (any further period of rest, they explained, 'is unlikely to result in permanent cure, and delay causes unnecessary suffering and possibly

54

a neurosis'). The operation, they had found, was safe – in no instance had any patient been made worse – and 'offers a high prospect of complete and lasting relief'; a verdict which was frequently to be echoed from other parts of the world.

Complaints blamed on the prolapsed disk

In the same issue of the *Lancet* there were two other papers dealing with back pain, one of them linking sciatica to prolapsed disks, the other attributing lumbago to the same cause. They had both still commonly been attributed to chills brought on by draughts or damp; now, in 1945, they were brought into the disk's catchment area. And three years later the author of the paper on lumbago, James Cyriax – a nephew of Edgar, and Mennell's assistant at St Thomas's – went further, laying claim to fibrositis, too. It had been in general use for unidentifiable pains in the back, and elsewhere. Its existence, Cyriax observed, was 'affirmed by most clinicians, denied by most pathologists'; as nothing could be found to account for it, the symptoms were under suspicion. Cyriax agreed with the pathologists; fibrositis was an imaginary disease. The term, he recalled, had been coined by Sir William Gowers early in the century, in an attempt to account for the pain by attributing it to inflammatory changes in the fibrous structure of the spinal musculature: so sciatica was 'primarily an affection of the fibrous sheath of the nerve'. For want of anything to put in its place, Gowers' hypothesis had retained acceptance. There was nothing the matter with the spinal muscles, Cyriax insisted. They went into spasm, certainly; but the fact that they did so 'provides a strong indication that the muscles themselves are normal'. The muscles were only trying to protect the spine from the consequences of a misplaced fragment of disk.

To any doctor who had been telling his patients for years that they had fibrositis and that there was nothing to be done about it, Cyriax's dogmatism was irritating. Patients do not ordinarily see the *Lancet*, but so startling an assertion might be picked up by the popular press, and as doctors had had enough trouble with patients asking whether their lumbago or sciatica might be caused by a slipped disk, for fibrositis to be under the same suspicion was unwelcome. In the correspondence which followed, some doctors cast doubt on the idea, pointing out that the pains of fibrositis sufferers were often related to changes in the weather, which they were unlikely to be if disk trouble were responsible. But the trend towards the identification and re-classification of formerly non-specific symptoms like fibrositis was too strong. For a while, the disk acquired what almost amounted to a diagnostic monopoly over backache, where no other specific cause could be traced.

Few orthopedic surgeons had much experience of spinal surgery; but this was territory which could also be claimed by the neurosurgeons. The spinal vertebrae and muscles, after all, were only the hollow mast, and its supporting stays. What was important was their content, virtually an extension of the human brain. If a disk were pressing on a nerve, that was the neurosurgeon's business; and in the United States he promptly proceeded to make it big business.

A surgical bonanza

It is interesting, even if profitless, to speculate how far it was the notion of a 'slipped disk' which was responsible for the popularity of the operation. 'The public are attracted by a new term', J. R. Armstrong observed in his *Lumbar Disc Lesions* (orthopedists had by this time quietly appropriated 'lesion' for their own purposes, after mocking for so long the osteopaths for their use of it); 'patients who ten years ago took their "lumbago" or "fibrositis" for granted, and in silence, now gossip with some pride of their "slipped disc" '.

No longer did people have to blame themselves for having sat on a cold seat, or failing to take a hot bath after getting caught out in the rain. Even more important, no longer did they have to make the feeble-sounding excuse of 'backache' for not going to work. A slipped disk was gratifying to the patient because it showed the pain was physical, not imaginary or neurotic; and satisfying to the doctor, because it was organic, not 'functional'. And so there opened up the prospect, quickly fulfilled, of a surgical bonanza almost comparable to that which had been provided by focal sepsis. How many operations were undertaken is impossible to calculate with any accuracy; but Dr Arno Sollmann, lecturing to the International Federation of Manual Medicine in 1968, estimated that 20 years earlier as many as two out of every three cases of lower back pain or sciatica were operated upon.

For a time, all appeared to go well. 'We hold the view', Burns and Young wrote from St George's Hospital in 1947, 'that nearly all recurrent attacks of backache, and many cases of chronic backache, are due to disc lesions'; the rational treatment, they asserted, was an operation, which was free from risk, and would provide a cure in nearly every case. The 1949 edition of a standard orthopedic textbook, describing the operation (the disk, it was explained, was 'cleared out with a sharp spoon') went so far as to claim that it was the only form of treatment which held out any prospect of a cure for lumbar back pain, or even of improvement. As late as 1959 the *American Journal of Surgery* carried an article describing how a group of surgeons in Portland, Oregon, had been treating 'prolapsed' (the term the profession had eventually settled on, to get away from 'slipped') disks for 20 years, using surgery where they thought it desirable, scooping out the pulp and, where indicated, fusing the spinal vertebrae above and below; and four out of five of their nine hundred or so patients had had good or excellent results from the operation.

Some orthopedists, though, had been voicing their misgivings. In 1949 A. G. Timbrell Fisher, a former Hunterian Professor at The Royal College of Surgeons, though welcoming the discovery of the relationship between backache and disk, warned that operations in some clinics were already assuming 'heroic proportions', in spite of the fact that insufficient time had elapsed to see whether the results were really so satisfactory as had been claimed; and eventually indications began to appear that they were not.

Doubts and reservations

It is at this stage that the researcher into the story of slipped disk surgery finds himself in difficulties, because the chief indication in the medical journals that all is not well is the absence of papers presenting statistics confirming the effectiveness of the operation. But there was one notorious indicator of impending doom: warnings about the importance of selecting the right cases on which to operate – a sure sign that some surgeons had been selecting the wrong cases. Medical journals, however, rarely contain papers showing a mounting proportion of failures of an operation. The reason is obvious: no surgeon is going to win any kudos, except for misguided honesty, in such circumstances. And his patients, if they hear about his failure rate, are likely to be extremely angry at the thought that they may have contributed to it – having been assured (as they commonly were) that the operation would end their suffering. At some point, they would complain, the surgeon must have seen that he was not getting good results. Why had he not stopped there and then?

Doubtless he often had. Or he might have gone on for a time, trying to be more selective in his choice of patients on whom to operate. But eventually he would abandon the procedure. So the number of operations has declined. 'Generally-speaking,' the New York surgeon, Lawrence Galton observes in his *The Patient's Guide to Surgery*, 'disk operations do not cure backaches'. Surgery is indicated only if all other methods have failed, and not necessarily even then.

One of the reasons for declining confidence in surgery for slipped disks has been the difficulty of diagnosing them. Disks tend to rupture on the wrong side of the spine for detection by 'feel'; and the damage does not show up on x-rays. For a time it was assumed that, lacking their shock absorber, the vertebrae above and below would shift towards each other, and that this would reveal itself in x-ray pictures. But it has proved an erratic aid. Sometimes they do not come together; sometimes they come together, but without damage to the disk – and without pain. In general, in fact, disorders of the spine, which appeared to offer radiology its greatest opportunity, have proved the most elusive to diagnose.

It has consequently often been deemed necessary to operate for the purposes of exploration; and surgery of this kind, too, has had some disconcerting lessons. Surgeons have been surprised to find that what had seemed clear-cut prolapsed disk cases have turned out to show no sign of prolapse; or, what can be even more puzzling, disks are found which appear to be in a lamentable condition but which have caused the patients little pain, or none at all ('the amount of pain does not seem to be proportional', the Manchester orthopedist John Charnley admitted in a letter to the *Lancet* in 1958, 'to the amount of organic change visible in the disk'). As, however, the proportion of cases where a prolapsed disk has been blamed, where no prolapsed disk has been found, is not ordinarily stated in a surgeon's papers on his work – not, at least, when they are published – it is impossible to gauge how many cases have been wrongly diagnosed.

What happens when a disk 'slips'?

Surprising though it may seem, too, in view of the tens of thousands of disks which have been dealt with by surgery, or examined in pathology departments and dissecting rooms, there remains considerable difference of opinion as to what actually happens when a disk slips. Almost the only point of agreement is that it does *not* slip: not, that is, in the sense of sliding right out from its position between the vertebrae. This it cannot do. But precisely *what* it does, and why what it does should sometimes, but not always, cause pain, has yet to be unequivocally established.

According to the Arthritis and Rheumatism Council's *Lumbar Disc Disorders*, a portion of the disk becomes damaged and bulges, or protrudes, usually in towards the spinal cord. As there is a strong ligament in its way, it deviates to one side where it may, and often does, press on one of the nerve roots which emerge from the spinal cord, causing the victim pain not only in his back but along the path of the nerve, in his arms or legs. 'A portion of the disk', however, is vague; perhaps deliberately so, as one of the unsettled issues happens to be about which portion is responsible. The Consumers' Association's *Avoiding Back Trouble* is more explicit. What happens, it says, is that if the fibrous layers – the cushion cover – which surround the pulpy nucleus begin to degenerate, small ruptures may appear through which the pulp can begin to escape. When an abnormal strain is put on a disk in this condition, it may cause a prolapse, in the form of 'a major rupture, or herniation, of material from the nucleus'.

Other authorities, however, are inclined to doubt whether it is the pulpy nucleus which is commonly responsible. James Cyriax puts the blame more on torn or displaced fragments of cartilage – not an academic distinction, he insists, as a different type of treatment is required if the pulpy nucleus is responsible: it needs to be 'sucked back by traction'. Most orthodox surgeons, though they would agree with Cyriax that manipulation does not help where the pulp has herniated through the covering, dismiss the idea that it can be sucked back by traction as fantasy; at best, they feel, the pulp may work its own way back, by some as yet not understood process.

The 'slipped disk', then, is not specific; nor, if it were, would any particular treatment automatically be indicated. And as it happens, there is no longer any confidence in the assumption that disks are the main cause – or even a common cause. Although Cyriax may maintain that disk trouble is 'all but universal', most orthopedists now feel that its incidence has been ludicrously exaggerated. 'Contrary to what many people believe, the trouble isn't anywhere near the commonest cause of back pain', David Delvin asserts. 'Some experts think it causes only about five to seven per cent of all cases of low backache'. A few have put the proportion even lower: a Milwaukee surgeon, Donald Thatcher, who investigated a series of

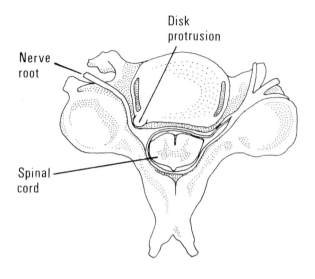

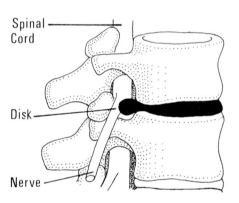

(Top) In this front view of a cervical disk the nerve root is shown to be compressed by the disk; (below) a side view of a disk where a nerve is 'trapped'. Today many authorities believe that the prolapsed disk as a cause of back pain has been grossly exaggerated.

100 unselected patients with backache, reported in the *American Journal of Surgery* in 1959 that only three had prolapsed disks.

There is now much more willingness to accept that ligament trouble may be responsible. Even Ronald Barbor, for years Cyriax's assistant at St Thomas's, has swung over to the view that backache is often due to this cause. By far the majority of backaches, according to Galton in his *The Patient's Guide to Surgery*, 'are the result of weak musculature'. 'Most of the time', Delvin agrees, 'when something gives, it is the muscle fibres or ligaments or tendons, not the spine'. One ingenious suggestion has been that tendon displacement, by causing a muscle spasm, may pull the vertebrae together, in the process actually producing a disk protrusion. And although other authorities refuse to credit that the muscles are to blame it is obvious that, as Crawford Adams observes in his *Outline of Orthopedics*, the diagnosis of disk prolapse 'is presumptive, and never unequivocal (unless confirmed at operation)'. Adams is referring to the diagnosis of disk prolapse in cases of neck pain; but the comment could well be extended to apply to backache in general, apart from those few cases which x-rays and other diagnostic aids show to be actual diseases of the spine.

For a time it was hoped that myelography – the use of an injection into the spinal cavity of an opaque liquid which would show up on x-rays, and reveal the presence of a protruding disk – would prove of greater assistance than straight x-rays had done. As long ago as the 1940s, admittedly, it was pronounced 'discarded as unreliable', in an orthopedic textbook – its unreliability not being confined to the difficulty of interpreting the information provided: botched injections had been too common, and a search through the medical journals in 1953 revealed over 50 cases of spinal damage suffered as a result of lumbar puncture. As in some of them the damage had not been recognized until months later, it seems likely that there were many more.

The use of myelography has nevertheless continued, as the 1977 *Manual of Acute Orthopedic Therapeutics* reveals. The authors, two Boston surgeons, warn that even when the findings are negative, they do not rule out disk prolapse, because the interpretation of them is subjective and 'fraught with many possible technical errors' – a depressing indication that such errors have been revealed by unnecessary surgery, because as a rule that is the only way they ever are revealed. They also add the even more sinister comment: a lumbar myelogram 'may not be a benign procedure'. And in Britain, although a questionnaire circulated to orthopedic surgeons and neurosurgeons by David Le Vay in 1967 elicited that myelography had gone out of favour, it has recently come back into fashion again – such is the anxiety for more reliable diagnostic techniques. But it has not, as yet, led to any increase in the proportion of cases considered suitable for surgery.

Where surgery is resorted to, it may take the form of simple removal of a disk; but this can involve laminectomy – removal of part of a vertebra; and sometimes 'fusion' of two adjacent vertebrae – effecting a junction between them of a kind which will enable the bone cells to get to work, in the same way as they do to mend a fracture, but which in the case of the spine means that the two vertebrae are converted into one. Like everything else in connection with disks, the value of fusion has often been questioned; but in last resort cases, where there is no other way in which the pain or other symptoms can be relieved, laminectomy and fusion appear to be reasonably effective and safe.

DRUG TREATMENT

You can take it, then, that unless you are unlucky enough to fall into the hands of a neurosurgeon who has decided that he has found, or is going to invent, a form of operation which works – and there are always a few of them, moved by visions of fame and fortune, and perhaps a Nobel Prize – an operation is not going to be recommended unless your condition becomes desperate. But it will also have occurred to you that periodically, over the past few years, there have been stories of new wonder drugs being marketed, some of them specifically for backache. Surely some of them must be available, and worth trying?

The story of drug treatment for back pain, and indeed for rheumatic-type disorders of all kinds, is even more depressing than the story of surgery. The honeymoon with cortisone was brief. It galvanized patients, but at the cost of superseding their self-regulatory hormonal system; once a patient was on cortisone he sometimes could not be taken off it without dire results. This might have been tolerated as a small price to pay to keep him up and about and enjoying life. But patients on cortisone too often found life hell. It produced as repellent a set of side-effects as any drug in history.

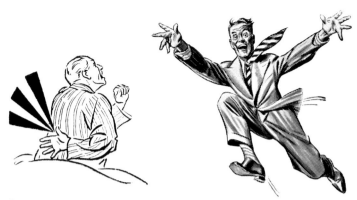

Plagued by Backache

until he started Kruschen Salts: Says:
'The Early Morning Dose Is My Salvation'

Claims of miraculous over-night 'cures' are never made for Kruschen. But it has been plainly stated in the past—and let it be just as plainly stated again to-day—that backache does yield to the *regular* daily dose of Kruschen Salts. Here is a one-time sufferer from backache who writes :—'*After seven days on Kruschen I felt better—could give a cheery good-morning without a special effort.*' Read his letter :—

'*It is with extreme gratitude that I write you after taking Kruschen Salts. The freshness with which one commences the day's work nowadays after having suffered from kidney trouble for years, is perfectly marvellous and well worth recording. I am 57 and my early morning dose of Kruschen is my salvation. I had continuous backache for four years, and looked on the black side of everything. After seven days on Kruschen I felt better—could immediately get up and dress and give a cheery good-morning without a special effort. At first I took 'enough to cover a sixpence' three times a day for seven days. I now need only take the morning dose.*'

Dec. 17, 1936. *J. T., Kensington, W.14.*

Pains in the back mean poisons in the blood—poisonous waste products which tired kidneys are failing to filter from the system. When these poisons settle in the regions around the kidneys they inflame the tissues and cause those excruciating pains. The six salts in Kruschen coax your kidneys back to healthy, normal action, so that not a particle of poisonous waste matter remains unexpelled. Your inside is thus kept clean and serene. You experience joyous relief from those old, dragging kidney pains. Then you can prevent the possibility of a relapse by continuing the tiny, tasteless pinch of Kruschen crystals in your morning cup of tea.

Take as much as will cover a sixpence every morning

Kruschen Salts

"Tasteless in Tea"

Every chemist sells Kruschen in 6d., 1/- and 1/9 bottles. Take as much as will cover a sixpence every morning. A 1/9 bottle lasts three months.

The Kruschen Salts advertisements were a familiar feature of newspapers in the Thirties; some sufferers still put their trust in this product today.
Courtesy, Ashe Laboratories

Not only were there the headaches, the dry mouth and the skin eruptions which are the common accompaniment of treatment with powerful drugs: the collapse of the patients' self-regulatory systems created the symptoms of endocrine imbalance: thin patients grew fat, and moon-faced; women and children grew facial hair. Resistance to infection, too, was lowered, so that people being treated were an easy prey to germs. And in some cases, cortisone unhinged the mind.

The drug companies hastily began to look for a replacement; and in 1955 they came up with a derivative, the corticosteroids. They were marketed as being as effective as cortisone, but safe. The side-effects certainly seemed less ugly; and for a time, all went well. But then an Australian doctor, Michael Kelly of the Melbourne Institute of Rheumatology, began to have doubts. After some unfortunate experiences with patients on cortisone he had switched to a steroid and, as he was later ruefully to recall, 'my critical faculties were dimmed'. Two years later, a patient admitted to him that she had had a mental breakdown after taking the drug. This disturbed him, and he decided to follow up what had happened to the 60 patients for whom he had prescribed steroids. To his horror, he found that six of them had died, one in a psychotic state, another in convulsions. He had not known sooner, because nobody had thought to connect their deaths with the drug.

A search through the medical literature left him in no doubt that his was not an isolated experience. Fatalities had all too frequently been reported. The effects were even worse, in fact, than he had feared. Certain disorders of bone and tissue, which had been given the name of collagen diseases, had been treated with steroids. Investigating, he found that the symptoms commonly attributed to collagen disease appeared to be the symptoms of steroid poisoning; and in 1963 he produced a list of examples, taken from medical journals all over the world, of the way in which patients were dying during or after steroid treatment – all the more distressing in that fatalities had rarely been reported from the disorders, including backache, for which the drugs were being prescribed.

In the meantime, however, drug companies had again spun the wheel in their game of molecular roulette, designed to produce a new type of steroid which could be marketed as safe: and in 1958 Merck presented Decadron, the promotion slogan claiming it had 'no steroid side-effects'. It captured a quarter of the American market in drugs for rheumatic disorders before independent trials disclosed that it *had* side-effects no different from its predecessors; and the President of Merck, John T. Connor, was compelled to apologize. He excused himself on the ground that the slogan had been intended only for use in countries to which Decadron was being exported, Britain among them (presumably it was for his services in this field that Connor was later to be elevated to Lyndon Johnson's cabinet, as Secretary of Commerce).

The next market-catcher was indomethacin, marketed as 'anti-inflammatory and analgesic' the promotion stressing the drug's effectiveness and safety in cases of lower back pain. It had not been long on the market when L. Meyler's survey of iatrogenic disorders – symptoms which arise from the treatment rather than from the disease – revealed that the side-effects were just as unpleasant as they had been from the earlier cortisone derivatives. In fact they appeared to be worse; but it might charitably be contended that this was only because doctors were by this time more alert to the hazards, and quicker to report them. The Canadian Food and Drug Directorate, worried by the number of deaths associated with treatment with indomethacin, sent out a warning letter to all doctors; and the United States Food and Drug Administration shortly afterwards followed its example.

Had indomethacin been really effective in removing inflammation and sparing pain, the continued willingness of doctors to prescribe it for patients crippled by backache, while warning them of the risk of side-effects, would have been understandable. But in 1967 two Boston doctors, Robert S. Pinals and Sumner Frank, reported on a trial they had carried out with 24 patients, half of them being given aspirin, and the other half indomethacin. The trial was 'double-blind', neither patients nor investigators knowing which patients were receiving the aspirin and which the indomethacin; half-way through, the patients were switched from one to the other in a 'cross-over', so that it would be possible to detect how each patient reacted to each. When the experiment was complete (three patients having dropped out), and the results compared, it was found that seven patients had preferred the indomethacin, seven the aspirin, and the remaining seven had detected no difference, so that subjectively there was nothing to choose between their effects. On more objective tests, like grip strength, the score was six better on aspirin, five on indomethacin; the rest no better.

65

Silence on the side-effects

A similar trial in Britain, but with a placebo, a dummy drug, rather than aspirin as the control, produced even more damning evidence against indomethacin: the patients on the placebo did as well as the patients on the drug. And that, it seemed, was that. Surely doctors would not go on prescribing a drug which produced serious and sometimes lethal side-effects, if its results were no better than those obtainable with aspirin, or with a placebo? Doctors could, and did. Some of them might have preferred to use placebos, and perhaps occasionally did; but this could be risky, if they were found out. Some had patients who did not do well on aspirin, or suffered gastric trouble from it, or developed allergic reactions; with them, too, the temptation was to use indomethacin. In the United States, the Food and Drug Administration imposed stringent conditions on the promotion of the drug, insisting that all reported side-effects must be listed, and that such claims as that it 'extends the margin of safety in long-term management of arthritic disorders', that had been used in promotion must be dropped. In Britain, no such restraints were imposed. Merck were able to embark upon a protracted promotion campaign for their version of indomethacin with such slogans as 'Mobilise the "low-back-pain" patient with Indocid' (1972) and 'In pain, inflamed, immobile – "Indocid"' (1974). In neither of the campaigns, conducted in full-page advertisements in the medical journals, were side-effects so much as mentioned.

This pattern has continued. New 'anti-inflammatory' drugs, lavishly promoted as safer and more effective, are put on the market. Each one attracts doctors and patients, and early comments are very favourable. But when reports from clinical trials come in, they show it to be no better than its predecessors. A typical recent example has been Chymoral, promoted as anti-inflammatory for use in lumbar disk prolapse treatment. After a double-blind trial at Guy's Hospital in 1975, one group of patients being on the drug while the other was on a placebo, the investigators reported in *Rheumatology and Rehabilitation* that although the patients on the drug fared a little better than those on the dummy pill, the drug's value was 'at best marginal'. And because it did not clear up the symptoms sufficiently to render other treatment unnecessary, 'we must conclude that the drug is of negligible value in this disorder'.

Periodically, though, some new technique of administering anti-inflammatory drugs is tried which for a time raises hopes of a breakthrough, the latest to win glowing reports being injections outside the spinal casing, which have been claimed to be both effective and safe. Always the hope is that a way will be found to use them without risk to patients; but in view of the side-effects listed by A. B. Myles and J. R. Daly in their book on the subject in 1974, the prospects are not encouraging. They show little change from those reported after the initial trials with cortisone: muscle weakness, high blood pressure (described as 'benign', though the symptoms include irritability, headache and vomiting), cataract, increased susceptibility to infections (notably herpes and TB), retardation of growth in children, redistribution of body fat (including 'moon face') in adults, mood disorders ranging from insomnia to psychosis, and osteoporosis, in which the bones become porous or brittle. 'Unfortunately', the authors remark, 'the changes do not become obvious until the osteoporosis, which may take years to develop, is well advanced'. It may be, against all past experiences, that a way will be found to make the anti-inflammatory drugs safe, but their record does not encourage confidence.

A more promising recent development has been the treatment of ligament disorders with dextrose, described by Ronald Barbor in a paper on 'sclerosant therapy'. It is based on the recognition that 'when a ligament is injured, normally nature cures', by filtering blood into it, bearing the cells which help to repair fibrous tissue. Thirty years ago this gave G. S. Hackett, an American doctor, the notion that nature might be given a nudge if some substance were injected which would speed up the process; and after some experimenting it was found that dextrose, a natural constituent of blood and an energy giver, performed satisfactorily in this role. How satisfactorily the method works in practice, and whether there are any snags, must await the result of controlled trials. For the present, it remains broadly true that if your GP prescribes a newly-marketed anti-inflammatory drug for backache you should follow a safer prescription: change your GP.

'CONSERVATIVE TREATMENT'

The reason is simple. If your doctor has been keeping abreast of developments in the theory and practice of dealing with backache, he will know that if new anti-inflammatory drugs are prescribed at all, they should be administered only in a hospital, where the effects and the side-effects can be monitored. The overwhelming weight of informed opinion, as expressed in the medical journals (though not in their advertisements) is that if a patient is being treated at home no drugs should be taken, except mild pain-killers.

The *British Medical Journal* offers a guide to current orthodox attitudes in a series devoted to surveys of different syndromes; and in 1977 John A. Mathews presented one on backache. Significantly, Mathews is a rheumatologist. When lumbago, sciatica and fibrositis were traced to the spine the rheumatologists, in whose territory they had lain for so long, might have been expected to relinquish them to the orthopedists and neurosurgeons. But the rheumatologists held on to them, and have recently been making most of the running in connection with backache, even using it in the provinces for empire-building to secure an increase in the number of clinics devoted to rheumatic disorders around Britain. Where there is such a clinic, many GPs prefer to send backache patients to it rather than to an orthopedic clinic. Mathew's recommendations are unequivocal. Where backache is mechanical – where, that is, the cause is not some disease – 'recumbency and analgesics remain the basic treatment'; bed and aspirin.

The process by which the medical profession has been forced to adopt conservatism can be charted in successive editions of orthopedic textbooks. In 1952, when Armstrong's *Lumbar Disc Lesions* was first published, although it was still possible to present orthopedics as a dynamic, developing speciality, it was evident that the enthusiasm for surgery and drugs was wearing off. Soon, specialists who had been sceptical about the disk, and the treatment, were surfacing again. In the *British Medical Journal* in 1955 the Manchester orthopedist John Charnley bluntly asserted that for the great majority of patients with lower back pain, there was no cure; no treatment, even, except reassurance.

Charnley went further: if patients were pampered by being given so-called treatment, many of them would be back with another attack of chronic lumbago a year or so later. And when the second edition of Armstrong's book appeared, three years later, he had to admit that there had been little progress in the understanding of backache – an unusually frank admission, at that time, when important advances were being claimed in almost every other branch of medicine. Too often, he complained, both patient and doctor still demanded dramatic measures; from which it could be inferred that he himself had little faith in them. By 1965, when the third edition was published, he had even less. There had been no progress, he feared. All that the medical journals had to show on the subject was the 'almost incredible ignorance' displayed in their correspondence columns.

The extent of the hold which conservatism has come to exert in the treatment of backache is illustrated by *Lumbar Disc Disorders*, the handbook for patients prepared by the British Arthritis and Rheumatism Council. Such works tend to provide what is presumed to be a consensus of the best current medical opinion; and as there is no reason to think this an exception, it is reasonable to assume that it represents orthodoxy's considered views. If the symptoms do not quickly disappear, the recommendation is, stay in bed, if necessary for weeks, in the most comfortable position obtainable, taking whatever analgesics your doctor may prescribe. If, however, the symptoms are not severe enough to require rest in bed – or if improvement is too slow – traction may be recommended: gentle stretching of the spine by mechanical means, applied by a physiotherapist.

When, for some reason, rest in bed is not practicable, the back may be supported either by a plaster-of-paris jacket, or by a surgical corset, both of them designed as far as possible to immobilize that portion of the spine where the disk is giving trouble. Only if there is no remission of severe or disabling pain, or ominous signs of disorders in other parts of the body, such as the bladder, is an operation recommended. And that is all – apart from a recommendation to take gentle exercise to help restore strength, when the pain recedes, and to try to prevent any recurrence.

Conservative treatment, then, is not really treatment at all. It is based on the Hippocratic principle that if no positive form of clinical intervention has been found to work satisfactorily, the physician should let nature take her course, contenting himself with helping her as best he can by prescribing rest, a suitable diet, and any aids to recuperation, such as exercises, that may suggest themselves – and for the great majority of people who suffer from an attack of back pain, the method works: a 1972 survey in a British general practice showed that nearly half were up and about within a week. Leaving it to Nature's healing power, however, does not now happen to be clinically fashionable either with doctors, who feel a little ashamed of being unable to do anything positive, or with patients, who have been conditioned in recent years to assume that medical science has the answers. So the convention has been established that patients should be encouraged to believe that they are having treatment; and 'conservative' happens to be a good, safe way of describing it.

It can, of course, be submitted that even if bed (or corsets) and aspirin do not constitute treatment, the traction and the physio-therapy do. But these are precisely the elements least highly re-garded by the rheumatologists and orthopedists, many of whom regard massage, radiant heat and so on as, at best, reassurance for the patient; perhaps providing him also with temporary relief, but doing nothing to promote his recovery. As for traction, Mathews evidently has reservations about its effectiveness; and other autho-rities actively disapprove of it. Armstrong goes further: all its

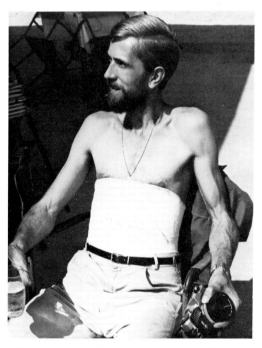

Plaster, first used in the 1870s for the treatment of back pain, still has its place in conservative treatment today; this patient, seen here relaxing in the sun, suffered an acute attack of backache during his overland journey from London to Calcutta.
Bill Coward: Barnabys

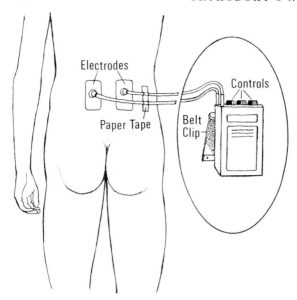

A battery-operated device available in the United States for relieving low back pain by means of electrodes taped to the back. *Courtesy, Dr Charles Burton, Sister Kenny Institute*

possible effects, he has claimed, 'are harmful in greater or lesser degree, depending on the force used'.

In the United States, admittedly, there is more reluctance to rely on conservatism, at least in neurosurgical centres. There has been a great deal of experimentation in pain-killing techniques: by electrodes, implanted in the spinal column; by the severing of nerves between vertebrae; and by 'dissolving' nerves through enzyme action. The results have been reported as very promising; but then, such results have always been reported as very promising – for a while. In any event, the nerve-killing approach does not offer any prospect for finding ways to prevent back pain. And although there is also a much greater readiness in the US to resort to surgery in the event of the patient's progress being slow – cynics suggest that this is not unconnected with the fact that a surgeon still makes a great deal of money out of the operation – orthodox treatment in general follows the same conservative principle.

71

2 Manipulative Therapy

You have accepted conservative treatment; and while you are lying in bed, or limping self-consciously around in a corset, the friend arrives – as he inevitably will, sooner or later – who has had the same trouble, or whose wife has had the same trouble, which has been cleared up in no time by manipulation. Why don't you try?

This may put you in a dilemma. Although manipulation of the spine is not rejected outright by orthodox medical opinion, a great many doctors are sceptical about it, and some are dead set against it. You may consequently find yourself having to decide whether or not to go against your doctor's advice. This is something which most of the writers of the standard works on backache beg you not to do even if his advice contradicts theirs – and they say it even in books sponsored by non-medical organizations, like *Avoiding Back Trouble*, produced by the Consumers' Association; 'If your doctor gives instructions that conflict directly or indirectly with what you read here', it insists, 'do what the doctor says'. 'Don't be surprised if what your doctor suggests is a little different from the advice we give here', David Delvin echoes, on behalf of the Back Pain Association. 'Please be guided by him, because he knows you and therefore should have a reasonable idea of what's best for you'.

A couple of pages later, however, Delvin goes on to give the game away: 'the really surprising thing about back pain', he admits, 'is that *we know so little about it*. Basically, that is the reason why it is so often difficult to treat'. Your doctor may know you, but the chances are that he will *not* have a reasonable idea, or any idea at all, of what's best for you if you get backache. Medical schools tend to concentrate on subjects which are well understood – or at least, where the area of uncertainty or disagreement is well defined. Students learn little about backache, apart from how to spot specific and easily diagnosed diseases. 'There is still an extraordinary gap in medical education', Arthur A. Michele, Professor and Chairman of the Department of Orthopedic Surgery at the New York Medical College, admits in his *You Don't Have to Ache*; and he quotes a comment made at a meeting of the American Medical Association that medical students devote only one per cent of their time to learning about muscles and bones, but 'suddenly we find ourselves in practice faced by patients, about eighty per cent of whom complain to us of some pain related to some part of the musculo-skeletal system'.

One reason is obvious. For the best part of a century medical students have been taught that sound clinical practice is based on accurate diagnosis. Their training has been, and still is, based on the assumption that the first duty of a doctor is to find what is the matter with the patient. Only when this is done, the assumption is, can he prescribe the appropriate remedies. And a glance at any orthopedic textbook reveals the care which has been lavished on this aspect of backache. Diseases of the spine – some named after the man who first discovered them, or first elucidated their symptoms: Pott's disease, spinal TB; a coarsening of the bones called after Paget – are listed and described in meticulous detail. But the abundance of detail is itself misleading. The tendency has been to devote space to diseases in proportion to what is known about them; and this has obscured the fact that Pott's and Paget's type of disease account for only a tiny fraction of everyday backache.

Orthopedists have done their best to make up for this by breaking down the symptoms of everyday backache into theoretically manageable, even if not clinically recognizable, segments. When terms like rheumatism and fibrositis are downgraded to colloquial status, their symptoms are re-named; divided and sub-divided, categorized and re-categorized by a process resembling the periodic revisions of managerial functions in the civil service or in industry, designed to promote greater efficiency, but endlessly confusing to the layman. Even doctors, if they are not orthopedic specialists, can usually be tripped up by the proliferation of terms anchored to 'spondylo' (of, or pertaining to, the vertebrae): spondylitis, spondyl-arthritis, spondylarthrosis, spondylosis, spondylopyosis, spondylo-syndesis, spondylolysis, and spondylolisthesis. But the identification of the particular 'spondylo' branch, or twig, from which the patient's symptoms hang, though gratifying to the doctor, is of small help to the patient, for frequently the diagnosis represents merely identification of the symptoms in jargon.

The label is not the cause

Curvature of the spine, for example, is lordosis if the bend is backwards; kyphosis if it is forwards; scoliosis if it is lateral. It is not unusual for a patient to be deluded into thinking that when one of these terms is used, it means the cause of his pain has been discovered. In many cases – as in the description of the various forms of curvature – pain is not even indicated. In others, the name simply is a convenient shorthand for the symptoms; and identification of the symptoms does not necessarily mean that a cause has been found, let alone a remedy.

Recently there has been a tendency to admit that the pursuit of identification in terms of pathology has been carried far past the point where it retains any clinical relevance. What doctor and patient need to know is whether the symptoms are treatable, and if so, how. Certain generalizations are again acceptable: for example, symptoms may be divided into 'mechanical' – slipped disks, muscle strains, degenerative changes – or 'inflammatory' – caused, perhaps by an infection. But the border territory here is ill-defined, and the causes of infections, if infections they are, not yet tracked down.

A more promising line is the classification of disorders into specific and non-specific. In the first group, Crawford Adams explains, 'diagnosis is positive, and rational treatment can be applied'; in the second 'diagnosis is largely a matter of conjecture, and treatment is empirical'. This is clearly a sensible notion; the trouble is that there is rarely agreement on what can, and what cannot, be regarded as specific. If orthopedists cannot even agree on the role of the slipped disk, one man's specificity can be another man's bunkum. Adams believes that rather more than half of backache cases are specific; but many other authorities feel the identifiable proportion is far lower. In one survey of 500 patients sent for investigation to a hospital in the south of England in the 1950s, only 27 could be diagnosed as having any specific disorder. 'The great majority of patients who complain of spinal pain', D. A. Brewerton – a consultant to the Royal National Orthopaedic Hospital in London – confirmed in 1973, 'cannot be classified or diagnosed accurately'.

Even if the diagnostic element were improved, the backache sufferer would not necessarily benefit. For years the orthodox assumption has been that when diagnosis becomes more accurate, as the Consumers' Association's *Avoiding Back Trouble* hopefully explains, 'treatment can be more logically designed'; with backache, it is not so much more logic as more inspiration that is needed. When Crawford Adams claims that where diagnosis is positive, rational treatment can be applied, it sounds reasonable; but when he comes to describe treatment 'rational' appears to mean 'appropriate', and the fact that a treatment is designated as appropriate does not necessarily mean that it is effective. In the single sentence which he devotes to the treatment of spinal rheumatoid arthritis, for example, Adams says that it should be on the lines which he has already recommended for the treatment of rheumatoid arthritis in general, earlier in the book. Turn back to that section, and you find yourself confronted with the blunt admission, 'the treatment of rheumatoid arthritis is unsatisfactory. No specific cure has been found'.

In general, then, it is fair to say that orthodoxy's pursuit of diagnostic certainties has been unrewarding. In backache, the idea that your doctor knows best is an illusion; as, indeed, GPs have increasingly been prepared to admit, at least in private (in an article in the *Daily Express* the columnist George Gale has perceptively remarked that the people who are most sceptical about modern medicine are those who know their doctor socially). And with the relaxation of the rules prohibiting doctors from referring patients to an unqualified practitioner, there has been a greater willingness to allow, even encourage, backache sufferers to try manipulative therapy from osteopaths or chiropractors.

Many people, however, feel safer if they are being treated by a qualified doctor, even if his methods are unorthodox; and in Britain, such doctors are not quite so rare as they are in the United States.

When the rheumatologist John A. Mathews told the readers of the *British Medical Journal* in 1977 that 'recumbency and analgesics remain the basic treatment for most mechanical spinal lesions', a correspondent wrote in to say that he 'must respectfully disagree' – and then went on to disagree far from respectfully. His patients, he claimed, usually complained that their pain was the worse with rest, eased by exercise; bed, he felt, was the worst possible treatment for anybody with postural or occupational backache. Another correspondent, dismissing the rationale behind conservative treatment as a 'gross oversimplification and misrepresentation', went on to

75

argue that the restoration of function in the joints was more important than 'restoring anatomy'. And these letters reflected the view of a minority of GPs, rheumatologists and orthopedists who, believing that the restoration of function is of importance, rely on manipulative therapy.

What is manipulation?

'Manipulation' has a variety of clinical, as well as colloquial, definitions: and attempts which have been made to clarify them, for

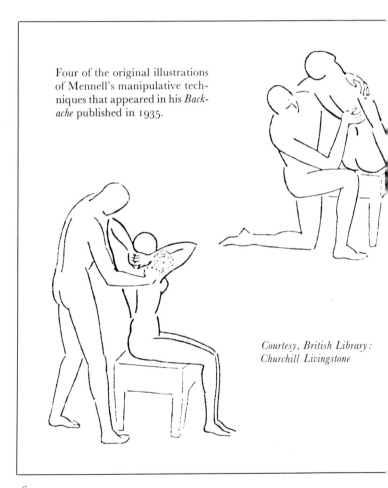

Four of the original illustrations of Mennell's manipulative techniques that appeared in his *Backache* published in 1935.

Courtesy, British Library: Churchill Livingstone

example by dividing it up into 'active' and 'passive' manipulation, have not proved satisfactory. It is usually distinguished from massage by the convention that massage deals with soft tissue, whereas manipulation deals with bone; but this distinction is blurred, for the obvious reason that things have to be done to the muscles to facilitate what is being done to the joints. And though the term manipulation is not generally used about actions taken for a specific clinical purpose like reducing a fracture or a dislocation, it can be applied to them, too.

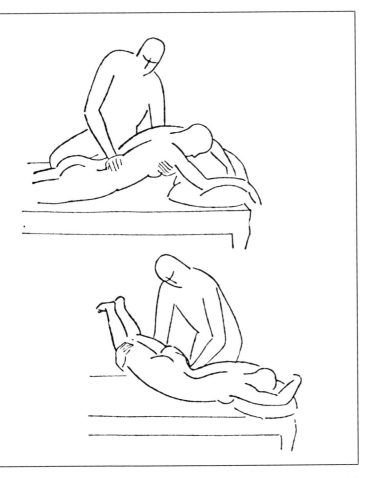

The term is most commonly employed, though, in two contexts; to denote the use of force to break down the adhesions that the body erects around joints which are out of place, to keep them from straying further; and to denote the use of pressure or force, which may vary from the lightest of touches to a smart, vigorous shove, to restore mobility of joints or vertebrae. There is no clear-cut distinction between this and physiotherapy: some physiotherapists employ manipulation, when they can. But ordinarily, physiotherapy is regarded as playing a supportive role to conservative treatment, its aim being to keep the patient's musculo-skeletal system in good trim against the day when he recovers from his back pain; whereas manipulation provides an alternative to conservatism. Although it can be used as an ally of conservatism, ready to be called upon when the time is considered ripe, most orthopedists think of manipulation as a rival: a pretender, hoping to oust conservatism from its throne. Most manipulators, too, do not regard themselves as being there to supplement orthodox treatment, as the physiotherapist does. Often they are aware that they are preachers of heresy.

The protagonist of manipulative therapy was James Cyriax, who has recently retired from his post at St Thomas's, but remains Visiting Professor in Orthopedic Medicine at the Rochester Medical Center, New York, and has founded an Institute in London to further his causes.

In the 1945 article in the *Lancet* in which he identified lumbago with prolapsed disk, Cyriax was still cautious, recommending conventional rest in bed for a few days, with 'gentle passive movements' to get the joints moving again. By 1948, however, he was advocating more positive manipulative treatment. For sciatica it was simply a matter of securing 'the reduction of the inter-articular displacement causing the symptoms' by manipulation of the vertebrae of the neck. In lumbago, too, he claimed about half the cases responded to manipulation, and most of the others to a local anesthetic.

Here, then, lay the possibility of the plaiting of the two strands which St Thomas's had brought together: the manipulative methods advocated and practised by Mennell, and those demonstrated by Barker (still living in the Channel Islands; honorary consultant to a hospital there). In 1948, too, manipulation received the backing of A. G. Timbrell Fisher, a distinguished orthopedic surgeon; in a new edition of a book on the subject, originally published in 1925, he lamented the medical profession's attitude, which 'savoured a little of apathy and indifference, or even of incredulity'; and which, he feared, was based on 'two hoary traditions' – that manipulation was unnecessary, and that it might have untoward consequences. Neither, he insisted, was true, provided the diagnosis was sound.

Timbrell Fisher's plea went unheard. Why risk a speculative diagnosis, which might be unsound, when opening up the patient's back could reveal precisely what was the matter? If a prolapsed disk were found, it could be dealt with. And if it were not disk trouble – if, say, some inflammatory condition of the joints were responsible – cortisone became available. So manipulation, never in favour, could be ignored.

An alternative to conservative treatment

With surgery and drugs losing favour, however, and with orthodoxy forced back into conservatism, Cyriax has had his opportunity. In *The Slipped Disc* (1970) he has listed the measures on which conservative treatment relies, and one by one demolished them. Rest in bed, he is prepared to concede, at least costs the National Health Service nothing; but it wastes the national resources. Its disadvantages for lumbago are manifold; it adversely affects patients, because it causes them unnecessary pain and disablement, and loss of earnings for longer than necessary; it wastes the doctor's time (and makes him look silly if the patient is subsequently cured by a lay manipulator); and it costs the community enormous sums in sickness benefit. Plaster jackets are no real help. Corsets have a bad name with patients. Most exercises are actually harmful; heat and massage, expensive and useless. Yet these are the measures universally adopted in Britain, 'despite the fact that they are manifestly futile, waste endless time, use scarce and expensive personnel and equipment, and predispose to neurosis'. In his younger days, Cyriax recalls, the treatment for lumbago was a belladonna plaster and aspirin, costing a few pence. 'In these enlightened and scientific days, equally valueless methods are employed, but all expensive in time or money, or both.'

In place of conservative treatment Cyriax offers his own brand of manipulation. His description is not easy to follow; but such descriptions never are. The commonest indication for manipulation, he believes, is 'a small fragment of disc lying displaced within a spinal joint' (elsewhere he claims that it is the *only* reason he knows for

79

manipulating a spinal joint, other than the couple at the top of the spine). The initial manipulative moves are those which, in the past, have been found to give good results; those which are least painful; and those which provide the manipulator with useful information. 'Working on the basis of trial, end-feel, and effect, the manipulator continues his series of manoeuvres, repeating or abandoning a particular technique on a basis of result and of end-feel.'

The strength of the manipulative movement depends on the circumstances; it can vary from a gentle push to 'a considerable, albeit controlled, thrust'; and the technique also varies according to the estimated size and position of the loose fragment. Sometimes it will be reduced, and the derangement corrected, even in advance of the manipulator's hopes; sometimes it will resist all efforts. But manipulation is all that is required, in most cases; though traction can be a help – traction being the only element in conservative treatment to meet with Cyriax's approval.

Believing as he has that provided a qualified practitioner makes the diagnosis, physiotherapists can be trained to do the actual manipulation, Cyriax has taught his methods to the physiotherapists who came through his Department in St Thomas's, as Mennell did before him; and doubtless many of them still follow his instructions, when they get the opportunity. But this training did not commend itself to the Chartered Society of Physiotherapy, dominated as it has been by orthodox thinking on the subject; and it is only recently that its resistance has begun to crumble. Physiotherapists, too, as medical auxiliaries, have only been permitted to give such treatment as the doctor in charge of the case orders, or at least sanctions. You cannot simply call for a physiotherapist, and ask for manipulative therapy – unless he is in private practice.

Medically qualified manipulators

Cyriax has tended to become a one-man band. His dogmatism has alienated him from many members of the organization formed by doctors interested in the subject: the British Association of Manipulative Medicine – usually called by the jocularly onomatopeic word its initials form, BAMM. Membership fluctuates between 200 and 300; medical qualification is a necessary prerequisite, but not manipulative qualification. Although courses are held for doctors who want to learn, they give no more than an introduction to the basic techniques.

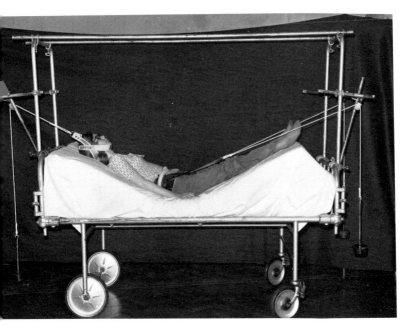

Spinal traction, one of the most ancient methods of treatment for backache, is still used today although its use remains controversial.
Courtesy, Robert Jones and Agnes Hunt Orthopaedic Hospital

Membership of BAMM does not entail adherence to any particular point of view about either the causes of backache, or what specific techniques to use in treatment. Many of its members take an almost diametrically opposed view to Cyriax's on the disk issue, contending that disks are responsible for an insignificant proportion of backache. Some believe in subluxations; some, like Alan Stoddard, author of a standard work on osteopathy, think in terms of vertebral segments which are immobile, relative to other segments – one analogy suggesting that the effect is comparable to what happens when a drawer in a chest of drawers jams, or judders when it is pushed in or pulled out; the pain coming from the protective muscle spasm. And individuals have theories of their own. The reasons for the pain are not of great importance in practice, however, because the type of manipulation used ordinarily depends less on the practitioner's assumptions about its cause, than on his experience of ways of relieving the pain.

According to Dr Burleigh Carson, Secretary General of the

81

International Federation of Manual Medicine, manipulation is a maneuver in which the joints are moved 'beyond their range of passive movement at the time'. The purpose is to restore normal mobility; 'it is best applied by slowly taking the joints to their extreme of passive movement and then applying a quick short arc thrust'. Guy Beauchamp, doyen of the medical manipulators in London, has described how a famous golfer once told him that the way to play the game was 'to hit the ball hard enough in the right direction', which struck him as being true for manipulation, too; 'it is a matter of making a movement in the right direction with adequate force; and in making that movement, the greatest force that is necessary is used through the shortest possible distance'. But it is not easy to describe the basic principles of manipulation. Even such standard works as Alan Stoddard's *Manual of Osteopathic Practice*, or *Douleurs d'origine vertébrale et traitements par manipulation* by Robert Maigne of the Hotel-Dieu in Paris – the most profusely and clearly illustrated of textbooks – find it hard to convey the action.

What the authors need, the impression often is, is one of those little books of action photographs which can be 'flipped' to show a golfer driving, or a footballer taking a penalty kick. A study of the standard works, however, soon shows that although there are differences of opinion, sometimes of a kind sufficient to arouse angry controversy, the differences of method are no greater, allowing for the much wider range of variations possible, than would be shown by flipping through books of photographs showing the swings of different professional golfers.

That manipulation can be extremely effective is beyond dispute. How effective it is, can perhaps best be demonstrated in a country like Britain where the manipulative method not merely has to compete against the prevailing orthodoxy: it has to compete on extremely unequal terms, because conservative treatment is free on the National Health Service. And on one thing both the medical manipulators and those who disparage them are agreed; that manipulative therapy, whether by the qualified doctor or the osteopath/chiropractor, is a flourishing, lucrative and expanding business.

But why, in that case, are there still so few manipulators who are qualified doctors? Why was Cyriax, in particular, with his forceful pen and his ready access by reason of his St Thomas's appointment (few BAMM members are attached to hospitals) to the columns of the medical journals, unable to win more converts to his cause?

Various reasons have been advanced, among them the fact that Cyriax was always by temperament a loner, finding it difficult to work in harmony with his allies in BAMM, and even more difficult to avoid giving mortal offence to orthodox orthopedists, whose conservative methods he dismisses with such disdain. But the chief responsibility lies with the medical schools. They are simply not geared to the introduction of a technique which requires a very different kind of qualification from any which the medical student is normally called upon to acquire. Manipulation cannot be taught, in the way that a straightforward surgical procedure can be taught. It can only be demonstrated, and learned by trial and error. In a flexible system of medical education, schools like that of Mennell at St Thomas's might spring up anywhere; but with a rigid system, devoted chiefly to the perfection of diagnostic techniques and treatments by the book, any therapy where diagnosis is not rooted in pathology, and any treatment which is based upon playing it by 'feel', is suspect. Manipulation can hope to secure admission only if its practitioners can prove conclusively that it works significantly better than orthodox conservative ways; and this, they have so far been unable to do.

The issue is not whether or not it can work *faster*; that is not in dispute, Burleigh Carson has given a table which shows the expectancy in cases where treatment is prescribed:

Treatment	Earliest improvement
Manipulation	seconds – 3 days
Sustained daily traction	2–3 weeks
Corset	1–3 months
Plaster jacket	1–3 months
Bed rest	2–6 weeks
Surgery	3 weeks–6 months

– figures which are broadly in line with those presented by orthodox rheumatologists and orthopedists. The orthodox, however, argue that although manipulation can give quick results, it does not work for everybody; and taking backache patients as a whole, its results in the long term are no better than those of conservative treatment.

83

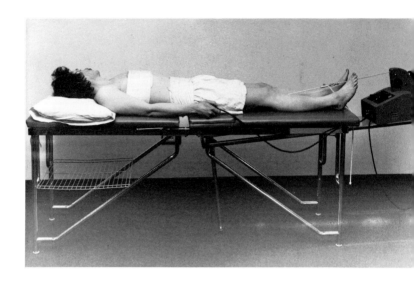

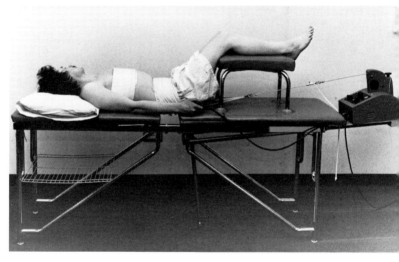

With this type of traction machine the pull in Kg, the time of pull in seconds and the rest period between pulls can be varied. The two positions are shown.
Courtesy, Institute of Orthopaedics, Royal National Orthopaedic Hospital

'The treatment works'

A number of attempts have been made to assess the effectiveness of manipulation in trials. In 1955 R. and S. Wilson, a British doctor and his physiotherapist, described how they had treated over 1,000 cases of low backache among industrial workers. More than half were attributed by the patient to an accident; and though the attribution, they found, could not be relied upon, it did not matter, as whether in the accident category or not, more than half had needed only one manipulation, and four-fifths had recovered after two. This could not be considered a controlled trial, the Wilsons admitted; but the results contrasted with the pain, boredom, anxiety, and loss of earnings suffered by those patients who were taking the conservative course: 'in our opinion, the treatment works'. That it works was also the opinion of Ronald Barbor whose results, which he presented in the correspondence which followed in the *B.M.J.*, had worked out at 57 per cent free of symptoms after one treatment; 75 per cent after two.

Three years later the *Lancet* published the results of a similar investigation by R. A. Bremner. It was unusual in that he admitted he had not used any standard manipulative technique: his method had been 'entirely empirical', designed to put the lumbar spine through its full range of movement while the patient was under an anesthetic. Ten per cent of the patients had been cured dramatically, and the great majority had benefited; it had been possible to discharge two-thirds of them after a single treatment. And though Bremner's description of his method sent a shudder through many practising manipulators, who feared that spinal manipulation under an anesthetic could be hazardous because the patient's defensive forces were doped, he received a pat on the back from Cyriax, who unloaded another set of statistics; of 370 patients treated in the mid-1950s, nearly half had recovered after one session, and 60 per cent after two. A follow-up over the subsequent three years, admittedly, had disclosed that over 40 per cent of those treated by manipulation had had a recurrence; but this was not entirely unexpected, as the assumption had been that some people have 'their' backs, as others have 'their' headaches. The figures would consequently need to be compared with the recurrence rate following conservative treatment, which might be no better.

Bremner's paper, however, gave the critics of manipulation their opportunity, which they gratefully accepted in the *Lancet*'s correspondence columns. Bremner's reasons for manipulation had 'no foundation in pathology', one of them pointed out, before posing three questions to the manipulator. What precisely, in anatomical terms, did he manipulate? How could he achieve a precise objective within the intricate spinal complex 'by a manoeuvre exercised on the exterior of the trunk?' And was it right that throughout the country, practitioners should manipulate for slipped disks when many of them had never even seen such a disk, at an operation? Another correspondent – ironically, from St Thomas's – argued that Bremner's work, though painstaking, was invalidated by the complete absence of controls in his series: it was just 'one more straw composed of clinical impressions'. And though a few weeks later a trial was reported in the *Lancet* in which miners with back trouble had been treated either conservatively – by immobilization, rest and plaster casts – or by mobilization with manipulation, and the patients who had been manipulated had fared significantly better, the advocates of controlled trials still did not feel that their full requirements had been met. The conditions had not been tight enough; they would require a trial planned in advance to eliminate possibility of bias creeping in.

Scepticism and disdain

This is something which has so far proved impossible to arrange. It is relatively easy to test the effects of a drug, by dividing the patients who are to be treated into two evenly matched groups, one getting the drug and the other getting placebos, with neither patients nor doctors knowing which group is getting which until after the trial has ended. But tests 'double blind' on this pattern cannot be carried out with manipulation, as the patients would know whether they were being manipulated or not – unless it was done under an anesthetic, and most manipulators regard this as unwise. So although from time to time individual doctors have written articles expressing their confidence in manipulation most standard works on the subject have continued to treat manipulation, if they discuss it at all, with reserve, if not with disdain. J. R. Armstrong devotes only four pages of his *Lumbar Disc Lesions* to manipulation, and they are largely devoted to warnings about its limitations and its hazards: because the results produced are 'not in any way under the control of the manipulator, and at best any improvement is essentially temporary', he believes that in treatment, manipulation has only a limited 'and probably evanescent place'. The latest volumes in the series *Recent Advances in*

Orthopaedics contain no reference to advances in manipulative therapy; they make no reference of any kind, in fact, to manipulation. And in the eighth edition of his orthopedic textbook Crawford Adams, though accepting that manipulation has a place in improving the range of movement of joints, does not even mention it as a possible treatment for prolapsed disk, or lumbago.

The scepticism of manipulation's critics, too, has recently appeared to receive reinforcement as the results of a multi-centre trial by D. M. C. Doran and D. J. Newell, sponsored by the British Association of Physical Medicine, and subsequently published in the *British Medical Journal*. Some 450 backache patients between the ages of 20 and 40 were distributed at random between four groups receiving, over a period of three weeks, either manipulation ('at the discretion of the manipulator') physiotherapy; bed and analgesics; or corsets. The results indicated that although the patients who were manipulated did rather better than the others (among whom there was little to choose), the difference was not statistically significant; certainly not sufficiently either to convert the critics of manipulation, or to give any satisfaction to its supporters.

But the results were in certain respects misleading. Two members of the British Association of Manipulative Medicine had been invited to serve on the committee monitoring the trial; but they resigned, as they explained in the correspondence following its publication, when they found that the Association had established criteria without consulting them which, they felt, biased the trial against manipulation. Ironically congratulating Doran and Newell for performing a public service by showing that manipulation had little effect 'when the cases are selected at random', Cyriax revealed the reason for the manipulators' objection. Randomization had been considered essential for the test on the ground that if the manipulator were permitted to select his patients, he would naturally choose those he considered to be most likely to respond to his treatment, which would mean that the results would not be applicable to the treatment of backache patients in general. But as Cyriax was implying, and as the great majority of manipulators would have agreed, the selection of suitable cases is an essential pre-condition of manipulative treatment (some would have added that it is also desirable for the patient to select himself, in the sense that it should be his decision – as in practice it usually is – to go to a manipulator).

The manipulators in the BAPM trial, who were not named, had

87

presumably decided that the technique would show results even if he were not permitted to select the patients: and in fact it did – but not within the strict terms of the investigation. As usual, in such trials, it had been agreed that the case histories of those patients who did not complete the course would not be included in the statistics. Of the seventy-odd patients who were in this category, 40 were on manipulation, and 26 of them stopped because they felt so much better that they did not need to continue treatment; a highly significant figure. To disregard them – or, for that matter, to disregard those who were being manipulated who discontinued treatment for other reasons – may have been deemed necessary to observe the protocol that has enmeshed such trials, but it was patently ridiculous from the point of view of assessing the value of manipulation.

Outcasts from the medical Establishment

The published results, Cyriax feared, would prove a deterrent to the introduction of manipulation as an orthodox technique. He was right. Even Delvin, who has some kind things to say about manipulation in *You and Your Back*, accepts that the trial showed there was 'little to choose' between it and conservative therapy; and whenever manipulation is advocated, there is likely to be a reminder, in a letter or in editorial comment, of the results of the BAPM trial. The attitude, and the reminders, will continue until a better designed trial is undertaken, and completed.

But it will take more than a controlled trial, however favourable its findings, to break down the prejudice within the profession against manipulation. The doctor who practises it, Cyriax has lamented, 'tends to become associated in his colleagues' minds with all sorts of dubious laymen'. How fierce orthodox prejudices have been is described by J. F. Bourdillon, in his book on manipulation published in 1970. As a medical student at Oxford he attended a meeting of the Osler Society, addressed by one of the most famous doctors of the age, who made what Bourdillon recalls as 'a deliberate attempt to brainwash his hearers against manipulation'; and later, as a student at St Thomas's, Bourdillon was 'strongly advised by the orthodox surgeons to have nothing to do with Mennell's department', because even within their own hospital, Mennell and Cyriax 'were considered to be little better than outcasts'. Bourdillon had strained his back in a motor-cycle accident, and the conservative treatment he received was ineffective; yet, as he wryly recalls, it was only after he had qualified, when patients with whom he had been unsuccessful 'were kind enough to let me know that subsequent visits to non-medically qualified manipulators had given satisfactory relief' that he began seriously to study manipulative theory and technique, and to evolve his own. But in this, Bourdillon has been exceptional. Most orthopedists – however dispassionately they may discuss manipulation, judiciously weighing its pros and cons – have an emotional prejudice against it, more intense than they are likely ever to realize, let alone admit. GPS are in general much less hostile, today, than they were even as recently as a decade ago; but there has been no great demand from them for manipulation to be included in medical training.

3 Osteopathy

If, then, you decide you would like to try what manipulation can do for your back, you may well feel compelled to shop around outside the profession. Your doctor may deplore this; but, as Cyriax has asked,

> Who created the lay manipulator? Alas, the doctors themselves, whose neglect of a simple method of treatment, practised with good results throughout the world for centuries, has forced sufferers to look outside the profession for simple manual measures. The patient cannot be blamed if, told that he has a spinal displacement, he seeks help from a manipulating layman when neither his own physician, nor the physiotherapist, nor the hospital consultant makes any move to put it back. Every family doctor, every medical officer in industry or the services, knows of this constant trickle to the layman. Yet a century of such awareness has not led to any visible steps to close such a conspicuous hiatus in the medical facilities available to the nation. Of all the maladies to which man is heir, it is only those amenable to medical manipulation for which our Health Service makes no appreciable provision . . .

So you ask your friends what you should do – and in all probability somebody has already volunteered the information; you should try an osteopath, or a chiropractor.

THE OSTEOPATH IN AMERICA

'An osteopath' or 'a chiropractor', though, are almost meaningless as definitions. For a start, there is a profound difference between the American and the European species; again, for historical reasons.

It happened that the American Medical Association was a much less powerful lobbying force, socially as well as politically, than the British Medical Association, partly because its members were so scattered, partly because the profession had taken longer to establish itself with the same strict rules and conventions that the British law allowed the General Medical Council to impose. But even more important, unqualified practitioners provided treatment in areas all over America where there were hardly any doctors; often no doctor at all, within emergency-call range. Any attempt by the profession to push laws through State legislatures discriminating against unqualified practitioners would run up against determined opposition. The profession, too, by its constant hammering away at the theme that osteopaths were not properly trained, drove them to reform their training schools. Investigating osteopathy on behalf of the Canadian government during the first world war Judge Hodgins reported that its whole character was changing; osteopaths generally were no longer adhering to Andrew Taylor Still's original tenets, but were determined to attain the same general clinical standards as doctors. As they began to do so, manipulation gradually became just one of their techniques, rather than *the* technique. But as doctors ordinarily did not manipulate at all, osteopaths were likely to pick up most backache cases.

As the osteopaths graduated to greater clinical – and legal – respectability, their 'hob-nailed-boot' place was taken up by chiropractors, using slightly different manipulative techniques; treating patients in a way which might often more closely resemble the methods used by the founder of osteopathy than the methods of some of the younger osteopaths, more conventionally trained. And the osteopaths, in their turn, reacted very much as the medical profession had reacted to them. Chiropractors, they complained, were charlatans and quacks masquerading under false colors – D. D. Palmer, they believed, had copied his technique from an osteopath, his differences of method having been designed simply to disguise the fact that he *had* copied it. Chiropractic, an osteopath complained in 1925, was 'the malignant tumor on the body of osteopathy'. In many States, particularly in California, the chiropractor was savagely persecuted, but he survived and began to flourish for much the same reasons as the osteopaths had earlier; he was providing treatment for farmers and villagers in outlying settlements where there were no doctors or osteopaths. And so the manipulative tradition survived. It became progressively more difficult for the profession to treat osteopaths as pariahs while they grew in number – there were about 13,000 in practice by the 1970s – and their hospitals – 300 of them – became familiar and respected. In most States, they began to enjoy a standing almost the same as a doctor's; in some, they were accepted by the profession *as* doctors.

The AMA vehemently opposed any such recognition, not so much from antipathy to manipulative treatment, though that existed too, but mainly on the familiar ground that osteopaths did not have adequate clinical training, so that however expert the technique, they might make disastrous mistakes such as manipulating a cancerous spine. But when in 1959 a committee of the AMA was set up to investigate osteopathy, and visited five of the osteopathic training colleges, its members found that the standards for entry and qualification were as high as in medical schools; that the teaching was better than in some; and that the osteopathy students actually had more hours of instruction than medical students.

By this time, according to the Committee's report, the only fundamental difference in principle between osteopathic and medical teaching lay 'in the emphasis placed upon the study of the musculo-skeletal system and the application of manipulative therapy'; but it went on to add, significantly, that 'the use of manipulative therapy is decreasing in colleges of osteopathy and is increasing in the orthopedic and physical medicine departments in medical schools'. The reason for this decline in the use of manipulation by osteopaths can be traced back to the 'wonder drug' era after the second world war, when disease after disease, it seemed, was being eliminated. It had earlier been possible for them to continue to believe that manipulation alone could treat diseases more effectively than the doctor could with his drugs, and many patients had felt that way too; but manipulation could not hope to compete with antibiotics. Osteopathy, however, was sufficiently well established in so many States that osteopaths were not put at a fatal disadvantage. They were allowed to prescribe drugs; and in the process, which inevitably tended to erode the distinction between them and doctors, they became more than ever determined to prove themselves the equal of doctors on the doctors' own terms. They have consequently since modified their earlier belief in manipulation as the main, let alone the sole, form of treatment; and although the chances are that an osteopath trained at one of the United States colleges will use manipulation much more readily, and more expertly, than an orthopedic surgeon, the differences between the two have every year been becoming less marked. And chiropractors have been moving in the same course, though they are not yet so far advanced along it.

THE OSTEOPATH IN BRITAIN

In Britain, osteopaths and chiropractors have everywhere had to compete with doctors. There was always a doctor, usually a hospital, within emergency call range; and if manipulation was required, there was the bone-setter. Osteopathy and chiropractic, therefore, did not develop indigenously, and until the 1920s were little known. But a few individuals went to America to investigate, trained there as osteopaths and came back to introduce the method into Britain; an osteopathic society was formed shortly before the first world war, and a training school in 1915; and in 1924 an anonymous writer in the *British Medical Journal* uttered a warning about a 'colossal system of pseudo-medical practice' which was creeping in. Although it had caused much trouble to the medical profession across the Atlantic, he wrote, Britain had been free from its adherents' incursions, but as there were indications that this immunity was coming to an end it would be as well for doctors to know about them. Osteopaths, he warned (and chiropractors, whom he dismissed as seemingly osteopaths under another name) rejected the bacteriological theory of disease, preferring to base their pathology on 'the science of vertebral subluxations', a science which he proceeded to ridicule: for if such subluxations existed anywhere but in osteopaths' imaginations, they would long ago have been demonstrated in the post-mortem room.

This was to become one of orthodoxy's main lines of criticism of osteopathy; another being that the training, particularly in diagnosis, was inadequate. But though these arguments sounded convincing to doctors, backache sufferers were apt to be more impressed by the actual results which were credited to osteopaths; and the demand led to the opening of the first clinic in London, with Bernard Shaw on hand to speak at the ceremony, echoing Paget by telling doctors that they should learn to manipulate. And by the 1930s, osteopaths had sufficiently established themselves for a Bill to be laid before the House of Commons by the young Robert Boothby to regularize their status by making it illegal for anybody to describe himself as an osteopath who had not undergone the prescribed training.

93

Private Members' Bills of this kind rarely get any further than the paper they are printed on, and the medical profession saw no reason for alarm, even when this one was brought up again in 1933 and 1934. But occasionally the House of Lords can be persuaded to accept a proposal which would stand no chance in the Commons, and in 1935, the Lords agreed to set up a Select Committee to investigate the subject. Two books, too, were published that year which intimated that orthodoxy could no longer rely on ridicule to demolish osteopathy's pretensions. *The Osteopathic Lesion*, by George Macdonald and W. Hargrave-Wilson, both doctors, confronted the profession on the issue which it had regarded as osteopathy's weakest point. There *was* such a thing as a spinal lesion, they insisted. It was essentially a strained joint, produced by either a strain, or an injury, or tension; and it had secondary effects, such as muscle spasm – and backache. The other work, though not concerned with osteopathy as such, was an even more serious threat to orthodoxy, because it was by James Mennell, Medical Officer of the Physio-therapy Department at St Thomas's Hospital, and it contained information which could only bring the osteopaths aid and comfort in their struggle for recognition.

Little progress had been made, Mennell pointed out in his book on the subject, in the understanding of backache, or in its treatment. The whole subject was among the most baffling in medicine; for backache was often complained of not just on its own, but in connection with other disorders, influenza, cancer, and even piles, gonorrhea, and smallpox. But if the nature and causes of backache were still not understood, there was one form of treatment, he had found, which was valuable; the manipulative technique he had learned from Dr John Deane of Boston, Mass., who had 'ploughed a lonely furrow', unable to convince his colleagues. Mennell knew, too, of doctors who, despairing of orthodox treatment, had gone to an unqualified practitioner, where their symptoms had been relieved. The time had come for them to practise manipulation, he felt; and he went on to describe and illustrate his technique.

Mennell's attitude was all the more disturbing to the orthodox in that it came from one of orthodoxy's citadels; and it was also all the more likely to hearten the osteopaths because it reached very similar conclusions to theirs by a different route. If medical science conceded that backache could be associated with piles or gonorrhea, was it not possible that Still's belief in the efficacy of manipulation of the spine

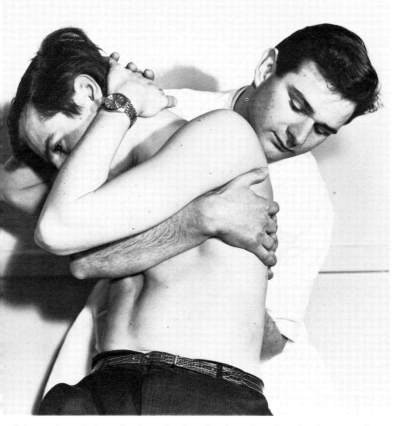

Diagnostic technique for investigating the thoracic spine. In the case of diagnosis, the osteopath aims to view 'the whole field of structural and functional changes which have disturbed the behaviour of any part or tissue of the body'.
Courtesy, British School of Osteopathy

for treating such diseases had some justification, after all? And though Mennell did not accept the existence of the osteopathic lesion, he came very close to it in his idea that soft parts might be 'nipped' by vertebrae.

The Establishment hits back

It was time, the medical Establishment – the Royal Colleges, the medical schools in the Universities, and the BMA – decided, to mount a counter-offensive. The Select Committee set up by the Lords was converted from an inquiry to elicit the facts about osteopathy into an inquisition, designed to expose the osteopaths as quacks and charlatans; with Sir William Jowett, who had been Attorney-General in the Ramsay Macdonald Government, as their prosecuting counsel.

Whether by luck or design, Jowett reserved his main forensic assault for J. Martin Littlejohn, founder and head of the British School of Osteopathy. Herbert Barker had cut a poor enough figure in court; Littlejohn's performance was far worse. As his non-medical qualifications were impeccable – he had higher degrees from Glasgow University – Jowett concentrated on casting suspicion on his clinical qualifications, insinuating that his claim to be 'MD (Dunham)' was meant to delude people into thinking he had qualified as a doctor through Durham University. Dunham was, in fact, a reputable homeopathic medical school in Chicago; but the shaken Littlejohn was unable to recall the names of any of his instructors, and was easily made to look both shifty and silly by judicious questions about whether osteopaths continued to accept the more esoteric view expressed by some of Still's followers. The British School of Osteopathy, too, could easily be shown to have inadequate facilities for the instruction of the students in such essential subjects as anatomy and physiology. Not surprisingly, the Select Committee's Report was scathing on the subject.

It was by no means so critical of osteopathy. Osteopaths, in fact, could infer from it that if they put their house (and their school) in order, their claim for recognition would be reconsidered. This was not at all to the medical Establishment's liking; and two young members of the British Medical Association's staff – Charles Hill (later to become the plummy-voiced Radio Doctor, later still to be one of Harold Macmillan's cabinet ministers, and eventually to be Chairman of the BBC) and H. C. Clegg, who was to become the editor of the *British Medical Journal* – between them produced a book, *What is Osteopathy?*, with the barely disguised intention of stripping it of any right to be taken seriously. There was no question, they blandly insisted, of the medical profession trying to kill off potential rivals, who might be offering the public a useful service. It was only trying to protect the public from people who could be shown through their own teachings to be peddling comically fallacious clinical doctrines.

To other doctors, the Hill/Clegg arguments, presented with an engaging air of 'we do not like to have to do this, but as it is our bounden duty, we might as well have some fun at the osteopath's expense!', appeared reasonable and persuasive. But a child could have pointed out the weakness of the illustration they used to prove that the medical profession had 'not been so stiff-necked as the lay public is apt to imagine' – the fact that St Bartholomew's Hospital had once employed a bone-setter, in the 17th century. In that case, the obvious reply was, why the resistance to Herbert Barker? Particularly as H. G. Wells, who allowed himself to be persuaded to contribute a foreword congratulating the authors for their 'intelligent explanation and exposure' of osteopathy, recalled that he himself had 'escaped from pain and lameness after a few minutes in Sir Herbert's competent and powerful hands'.

Wells' attitude was commonly encountered, at the time. Although he had himself benefited from going outside the profession, he was prepared to accept the orthodox line without troubling to investigate whether it was valid. And before osteopathy's reputation could recover, the second world war intervened, to be followed by the slipped disk mania, surgery and steroids. Disillusionment with these forms of treatment, however, brought custom back to the osteopaths (chiropractors were rare); by the late 1950s a few of them, like Stephen Ward, were running fashionable and lucrative practices; and unlike in the US, the great majority of the osteopath's patients came to him with backache, as they do to this day.

The osteopaths' caste system

There are osteopaths and osteopaths. In the eyes of the law – and of many doctors – they are all equal; but in their own eyes, some are more equal than others. The differences are not so much of technique, though they also exist, as of status. The rivalry is not on a horizontal plane, between different groups advocating different theories or methods; it is vertical – a caste system of a kind only the British could evolve, with a well-established pecking order.

Even leaving aside the members of the Osteopathic Medical Association, the small group of doctors who have had osteopathic training, there are no fewer than five categories of osteopath in Britain,

97

each reasonably secure in the assumption that they have the original message as handed down to Andrew Taylor Still from Mount Sinai. Most confident in that conviction are the members of the group centred on the London College of Osteopathy, who are differentiated from the rest in that they qualified in Kirksville or some other recognized training establishment in the United States. They think of themselves as, and call themselves, 'Dr'; and though the College until recently gave courses in manipulative therapy the students had to be doctors. Members of the College are even inclined to be patronizing about the British Association of Manipulative Medicine, some of whose members it trained. BAMM's training course, they feel, is hardly adequate. But they tend to feel more comfortable with doctors, from whom the great majority of their patients are referred, than with British-trained osteopaths who are not doctors.

The majority of osteopaths practising in Britain – about 300 – have qualified through the British School of Osteopathy. Following the humiliation of the 1935 inquiry, and on the advice of the Ministry of Health, a Register of Osteopaths was introduced on the model of the Medical Register, with a code designed to protect the public. Only those osteopaths who were admitted would be entitled to describe themselves as Member of the Register of Osteopaths – MRO; and disciplinary machinery was installed to make it possible to deal with members who failed to observe the code. At the same time, steps were taken to remedy the defects which the inquiry had found in the British School of Osteopathy and to bring it more into line with the equivalent US establishments; and this has since been accomplished.

The members of the College, however, held aloof, feeling that their training had been a cut above the School's; and this rift has still not been healed. The School's alumnae are consequently inclined to feel about the College much as a state-educated boy might feel about a private schoolboy; that he gives himself airs for reasons which are no longer relevant. At the same time, though, they have jealously withheld membership of the Register from a third group: the members of the British Naturopathic and Osteopathic Association – the BNOA.

Nature Cure, or naturopathy, is an eclectic form of therapy, derived from Hippocrates. If we lead a healthy life – fresh air, exercise, a balanced diet – the naturopaths believe, medicaments

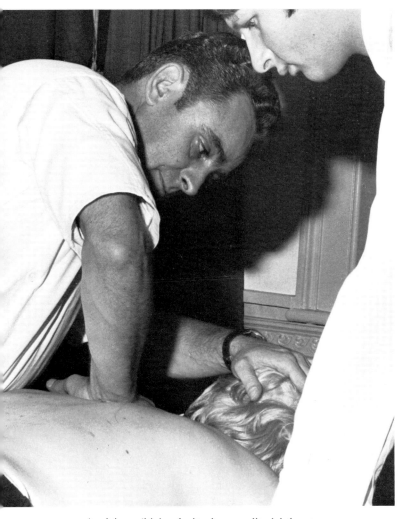

Applying a 'high velocity, low amplitude' thrust.
Courtesy, British School of Osteopathy

should be unnecessary; but as most of us do not lead healthy lives, aids like herbalism, homeopathy and manipulation (more recently, acupuncture) may be adopted. Originally most of the naturopath manipulators were self-taught, or had learned from bone-setters; but when the BNOA was founded, and a training school established, osteopathy became part of the curriculum, and the students when they qualified naturally wished to be admitted to the Register. But no: the British School of Osteopathy's influence was too strong. So the BNOA osteopaths remain a caste apart, with their own Register.

Recently they have split, into two sections. The osteopathically-orientated among them felt that the naturopathically-orientated were insufficiently interested in manipulation; so they took themselves off to form the Society of Osteopaths, with its headquarters at Maidstone, where an international school had earlier been set up to provide osteopaths for France and Belgium. But most of them have remained on the BNOA Register.

Lowest in the pecking order are those practitioners who profess and call themselves osteopaths, but have no formal qualifications – there being nothing in British law to stop anybody calling himself one, and practising as such, though he may have taught himself manipulation from a book, or picked it up from a bone-setter. There are also a few bone-setters, though they appear to be a disappearing breed. The last of them who could boast more than a local reputation was the remarkable Thomas Burke of Milltown Malbay in the County Clare, Ireland. 'Burke the bone-setter', as he was known throughout the county, used to offer to treat patients free so long as they were on the county electoral register, and would promise to vote for him at elections; and although the ballot was secret, which meant they did not need to keep the promise, he would get in – usually (the vote being by proportional representation) in the fifth and last seat to be declared. His electoral address in 1948 ran:

I once again appeal to the voters of every shade of politics and religion in Co. Clare. I now do so with very mixed feelings. You saw I had a tough time in 1944 to get even the fifth seat, though I had given the use of their limbs to people of every class in Co. Clare, without fee or reward . . . But now, when I want their No. 1 votes, I have to go on my knees and almost beg their votes off them. I do not at all think that treatment fair, especially when I thought that I had earned their votes and their gratitude . . .

As ever,
The same old Bonesetter
Thomas Burke

The electors heeded his plea; he scraped in once again. Clare doctors used to claim he was responsible for half the cripples in the county; but the triumphant appearance of Burke at the first meeting of the

Dail after the election (he had to attend and vote once, in order to qualify for his parliamentary stipend: though to avoid giving any of his electors' offence, he was careful not to vote again) suggests that the doctors were simply envious. He must have been a bone-setter of real talent.

'Instinct, practice and flair'

So there are the five categories: Collegers; MROS; BNOAS; members of the Society of Osteopaths; and plain, unadorned, unqualified osteopaths. If academic qualifications were all that counted, the osteopath's pecking order might serve as a rough guide to anybody seeking the best available practitioner. But apart from the fact that the academic standards of all the training establishments have been improving – and are going to improve even more rapidly, because the demands for places in them has been increasing, so that they can impose higher entry qualifications, and expect their output to be of higher quality – osteopathic manipulation does not, and cannot, depend for its success on the academic abilities of the students, or even the academic quality of their instruction. 'Burke the Bone-setter' was outstanding in Clare, as Barker was in London, not from qualifications but from a combination of instinct, practice and flair.

This is something which has frequently been illustrated in the newspapers – usually in the sports pages. A typical recent example has been the story of Gerry Francis, captain of the English football team. Playing in a league match in November 1975 Francis fell heavily on the base of his spine; and thereafter periodically it pained him until, the following summer, he was unable to walk, A trapped sciatic nerve was diagnosed by an orthopedic surgeon; but attempts to free it by orthodox means were unsuccessful. Next, a neurologist – Sir Roger Bannister – the breaker of the four-minute mile – had a try. After a spell of conservative treatment had had no effect, a myelogram was prescribed, which made Francis feel much worse. He was recommended to go to a neurosurgeon; but perhaps luckily for him the man had a waiting list and in the meantime Francis met the Secretary of the BNOA, Terry Moule; and Moule bet Francis a dinner that he could cure him in a couple of weeks. In fact, the treatment did not need to continue for so long: after four sessions, in ten days, Francis was ready to play football again.

To an osteopathic purist, Moule would be regarded with some suspicion, believing as he does that manipulation is no more than an adjunct to nature cure. Very possibly, too, his success with Francis was due to, or at least helped by, rapport: it would not necessarily have worked with another footballer. But such accounts are too common to be dismissed simply as luck, or coincidence. Football teams, as Moule points out, often have doctors who are not really well versed in spinal injuries; whereas Moule himself did a course which, even if it did not go over all the ground covered by the medical student, concentrated much more on such problems as backache, and how to treat it. And on top of that he has had some 13 years of experience.

If you want manipulative treatment, then, it is not simply a matter of looking up the yellow pages and telephoning the nearest osteopath in the expectation that he will be suitably qualified. Even if he is qualified, the suitability will be a matter of opinion; to those above him in the pecking order his credentials may be suspect. And within the medical profession, the proliferation of those credentials – MRO, MBNOA and so on – is looked on as clinical climbing, giving those who acquire them a sense of satisfaction, but impressing everybody else only as pretentious, perhaps bogus. Critics of osteopathy commonly argue that until the various osteopathic organizations get together, settle their differences, merge their training schools (or at least their curriculum), and introduce a single meaningful qualification, they cannot expect to be taken seriously. When they have put their house in order, it will be time enough to consider what their status should be; for example, whether they should be brought within the National Health Service, and if so, in what role. Should they be the equivalent of doctors, or of auxiliaries; or should they be in some paramedical category of their own?

Paradoxically, however, the main reason for the divisions between the different groups of osteopaths is the anxiety of each group to *preserve* its credibility, with a view to improving osteopathy's status. Because the members of the London College, with their US training, felt themselves to be the equivalent of doctors, they assumed that if they were to win acceptance as such, they must not become identified with the British School – particularly after the battering it received from the Lords' Select Committee in 1935. That humiliation has made the members of the British School, in turn, the more reluctant to grant admission to the Register of Osteopaths to anybody who has not qualified through the School. The BNOA similarly feels bound to deny admission to unqualified manipulators, however highly thought of, who have applied to join. The initials, in short, reflect a genuine desire to preserve and improve standards.

Even if you can find to which group the nearest osteopath belongs, therefore, it will not provide you with any trustworthy indication of his abilities. But with manipulation, in any case, no conceivable system of qualifications could provide it. This, it is coming to be realized, is the weakness in the American system. The graduating osteopath, other things being equal, is now as well qualified as the graduating doctor. But however well qualified he may be in medicine, can he manipulate? He will know the basic technique, certainly; but will he have the. . .

The knack? The flair? The art? All manipulators concede that there is an element in what they do which cannot be adequately demonstrated – because the students, watching, can see what is happening, but cannot feel what is happening – and which cannot be taught. Broadly speaking there are three categories of manipulator, comparable to three categories of students at art school. One lot will never learn to draw, in the simple sense of being able to produce a recognizable and reasonably accurate representation. The second group will be able to do just that. But only the members of the third group will be able to produce a work of art.

The osteopath as artist

In manipulation, though, the skill of the manipulator is only one element. The artist applies his brush to an inanimate canvas; the manipulator's hands are dealing with the bones and muscles of living people, who react not just to the hands, but to the manipulator, and to their own expectations and fears. Stephen Ward – the American-trained osteopath who built up a society practice in London before being offered up as a human sacrifice by that society, following the Profumo affair – used to say that he often knew whether his manipulation was going to work from the moment patients came into his consulting room. If there was no rapport, he had found – if he felt no instinctive feeling of sympathy with them – then he could fail even with what would have been relatively simple cases. If there was mutual rapport, he could work miracles; not, he insisted, too strong a term.

Most manipulators would agree. But most would be thinking of rapport in terms of the immediate physical consequence; in particular, relaxation. Yet the inducing of that relaxation, though it can be of great assistance, is only part of the story. Some very successful manipulators have the reputation of being ruthless, sadistic even. Herbert Barker was far from gentle; he assumed, like most bone-setters, that if for any reason an anesthetic was not to be used it was in the long run best for patients if he disposed of their adhesions in a single, often immediately painful thrust. His art, and that of all the great manipulators, consisted in his ability to gauge the precise force required for any thrust which he made, so there was no unnecessary pain. It was instinctive, on the first occasion when he set the dislocated elbow; and thereafter with practice it became instinctive in the same sense as a golfer's swing, or a cook's tossing of a pancake to bring it back upside down and lying flat on the frying pan.

What you will need, then – or at least, what you will wish to find – is a manipulator who is an artist, regardless of his qualifications. But here, only luck and knowledgeable friends can help you. If there is an osteopath practising locally whom somebody you trust swears by, that is your best hope: whatever initials he has after his name, or even if he has none.

You may find that your doctor is willing to help. Almost without exception, osteopaths now report a much greater readiness on the part of the profession to advise patients who do not respond to conservative treatment to try osteopathy, and the recent decision by the General Medical Council that a doctor may take this course

ANDY CAPP

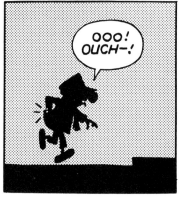
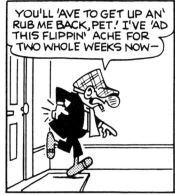

without risk of being struck off the Register, provided he keeps his patients under scrutiny, means that he can do so without risk. But a doctor is not necessarily a reliable source, because he tends to see the osteopath's failures – for the obvious reason that the osteopath's successes do not go back to their doctor; not at least, for backache. Some of the osteopath's failures may be disgruntled, particularly as they will have had to pay for his treatment; and doctors as a result sometimes get a one-sided picture. But an increasing number of general practitioners, at least, are being impressed by osteopathy's results. It is unusual to meet an osteopath who does not number a doctor or two among his patients (Stephen Ward had a member of the General Medical Council as one of his: it used to amuse him to speculate what would happen if a doctor were arraigned before the GMC for sending a patient to him).

THE OSTEOPATH'S OUTLOOK

What, then, can you expect, if you decide to try an osteopath?

Critics of osteopathy have no difficulty in showing that it does not have a coherent theory to account for backache; that its practitioners find great difficulty in describing precisely – or indeed, in any meaningful way – what they do; that in so far as their descriptions are comprehensible, they are often inconsistent, particularly in emphasis; and that on different sides of the Atlantic they

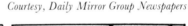

Courtesy, Daily Mirror Group Newspapers

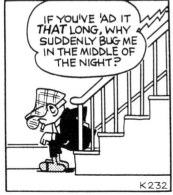

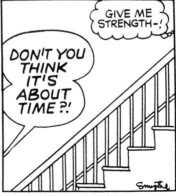

are so far apart in their attitudes that the term osteopathy has little meaning. Many osteopaths would agree. They claim, nevertheless, that there is a central tradition of theory and practice, deriving from Andrew Taylor Still, which has a basic coherence and consistency – much the same claim as Christians make for Christianity, when the diversity of their creeds and ceremonies is held against them.

To take diagnosis first. Osteopaths point out that there is a fundamental distinction between their way and orthodoxy's way; they do not put the emphasis on pathology. From the time a medical student embarks on his clinical training he is taught to look for the causes of the patients' symptoms in order to be able to pin the correct label on the disorders from which they are suffering. The examination which an osteopath conducts, as Audrey Smith has put it in her survey of the osteopathic diagnostic method, 'is NOT directed primarily at labelling a syndrome, but is aimed at viewing the whole field of structural and functional changes which have disturbed the behaviour of any part or tissue of the body'.

The reason is obvious: if, as osteopaths – those, at least, who subscribe to Still's ideas – believe, symptoms in any part of the body may be the result of a spinal derangement, there is no point in concentrating attention upon the symptoms. If a temperature gauge shows us that the car engine is overheating, we do not take the car in to a garage solely for work to be done on the gauge; we assume that something is probably amiss with the lubrication system. And as our bodies' lubrication systems – and much more beside; most of our information systems, too – are directed through the spine, the osteopath's primary concern is to find whether some spinal lesion is responsible for the pain, which will need to be corrected.

Again: 'lesion' is a loose term, and many osteopaths prefer 'derangement' – which, though as vague, comes nearer colloquially to Stoddard's definition, 'a condition of impaired mobility in an intervertebral joint'. Precisely what that condition is, and how it comes about, leaves them as uncertain as the orthopedic surgeon is over the slipped disk. Like the medical manipulators, some think in terms of subluxation (though that is a word the chiropractors have tended to make their own): a slight shift of position of one vertebra in relation to the next. Others talk of immobile vertebral segments; others believe that any anatomical explanation, however understandable in Still's time, needs modification: the trouble may be functional – as when we 'freeze' suddenly from fright.

Method of diagnosis

So far as patients are concerned, though, – and, indeed, so far as most osteopaths are concerned – the precise nature of the osteopathic lesion is relatively unimportant. What is really of importance, they insist, is to find where the trouble lies; a task ordinarily carried out by palpation, or diagnostic examination by the sense of touch.

Palpation is, admittedly, also used by orthopedists. Crawford Adams lists their four objectives: to find skin areas of unusual warmth or coldness, changes in the normal shape and outline of the bones, or changes in the muscles and tissues; and to plot the site of local tenderness. But these can all be regarded as quantitative. It would be theoretically possible, given sufficiently sophisticated instruments, to measure them. How far removed they are from osteopathic palpation can be gauged from an article by Rollin E. Becker of Dallas in the *Yearbook* of the American Academy of Osteopathy. Becker's argument is that as man is in total inter-relationship with the environment (another point, incidentally, which osteopaths have been increasingly emphasizing; the need for a holistic approach to health), terminology from all the natural sciences may legitimately be employed to describe the various aspects of the diagnostic touch including:

> compression, decompression, tensity, flaccidity, stress, drag, sag, strain, sprain, shock, contraction, expansion, torque, rotation, twitching, vibration, pulsation, mobility, motility, immobility, agitation, disturbance, oscillation, wabble, restriction, fullness, flatness, swelling, atrophy, dystrophy, irritability, strength, weakness, vigor, force, vitality, tone, power, potency, stillness, balance, fatigue fluctuation, and many others.

Many of these, admittedly, overlap; but they give some idea of the scope of the osteopath's diagnostic method. Yet at the same time, Becker's use of mainly mechanistic terms could convey a misleading impression. Osteopaths do not solemnly go through the motions of palpation, one by one, and make a note – say, on a scale of one to ten – of the degree of agitation, atrophy, and so on down to whatever 'wabble' they may find. They are trained, they explain, to consider all these things at the same time, so that if any differences from the norm are found, they will be a guide to the whereabouts of the lesion. If they are mechanistically-minded, they may present the analogy of a computer, programmed according to the information fed into it to print out certain relevant conclusions. Others simply claim that whatever the explanation may be, they find that with experience palpation provides them with guidance, along the lines pioneered by J. S. Denslow in the 1930s. An osteopath, he observed, would find when he examined patients that his hands tended to stop in certain places, almost of their own volition; a fault would be found there, almost as if experience was providing diagnosis as a conditioned reflex.

James Cyriax, sceptical of osteopathic pretensions, claims that although the findings from palpation may appear objective to lay manipulators, it is doubtful whether they would stand up to objective scrutiny. Again, though, osteopaths can reply that they are not concerned with precision or objectivity in their diagnoses; only with the lead it gives them to the appropriate manipulative treatment. There is nothing to suggest, after all, that Herbert Barker used diagnosis, in the academic sense of the word. He heard what the patient had to say, looked for and felt for certain signs, and applied the treatment which a combination of experience and hunch dictated to him. Many osteopaths, admittedly, would prefer to be able to make a conventional diagnosis, following the orthodox medical pattern, in order to be able to convince the profession that their treatment has a rational basis. But the lack of it is not destructive. They earn their livings, after all, not by telling patients what is the matter with their backs, but by putting them right.

How the osteopath works

To attempt to describe the techniques of osteopathic manipulation is a thankless task. Stripped to its bare essentials, in the brochure *The Osteopath – his work and training* put out by the British School of Osteopathy, the first stage is to relax the patient's muscles:

> This is not simply a matter of massage, but careful manipulation (stretching if necessary) of just those muscles which the osteopath's fingers tell him need treating. Next, he will move the affected joints, rhythmically easing them and firmly but gently encouraging more relaxation and movement at a very high velocity – a manoeuvre called the 'high velocity' thrust.

The thrust, their brochure notes, is the part which most impresses the patient, particularly as it may be a tearing sound and end with a 'click' – the noise which bone-setters used to tell their patients was the sound of the bone returning to its correct position. The tearing sound is taken to be the adhesions breaking down; what the 'click' is remains in dispute. But the high velocity method has in any case been receding into the background; gentler methods appear to be able to give the same results, without the risks that an over-enthusiastic thrust might entail. Most orthopedic surgeons have encountered cases where bones have been fractured by a lay manipulator – or claim they have; but in fact such cases appear to be extremely rare. The spine has incredible strength – as reports of the methods used to straighten it, from Hippocrates on, clearly demonstrate. And if lay manipulation were as lethal as orthopedists like to claim, the medical journals would endlessly be reporting coroners' verdicts to that effect as well as the subsequent legal actions; yet such reports are uncommon. Nevertheless osteopaths are coming to regard themselves not so much as thrusters, or even as re-positioners, of bones, but as releasers of the patient's own re-cuperative forces. And this can be not so much a matter of manipulation, in the accepted sense, as of . . . there is no word for it: tactility? Something of that kind.

This poses a problem for lay manipulators, whatever their allegiance. Again: they would like to prove that what they are doing is rational, as well as effective. But 'rational' has become so identified with 'explicable' in materialist terms that in order to impress, say, a committee of inquiry, even one which is not dominated by the medical profession, they must be able to document their procedures. They try: they produce works like *The Physiologic Basis of Osteopathic Medicine*, the outcome of a symposium on the subject held in New York in 1967. But the more they come to accept that manipulation is not just a set of formal actions, but also a way of establishing a form of rapport which enables the patient to do the adjusting, the less easy it becomes to justify their techniques on any mechanistic basis – or, rather, the less relevant their justifications sound in relation to what they actually do.

This is an issue which has concerned Irvin Korr, the metaphy-sician of osteopathy, in recent years. In his memorial lecture on the centenary of Andrew Taylor Still's 1874 osteopathic manifesto, Korr has listed some of the results of the research which has been done into the neurobiology of the spine which have been justifying osteopathic ideas. But there comes a point, he goes on, when it is impossible to squeeze osteopathic medicine into orthodoxy's incompatible and inimical framework, for to do so requires a distortion of the osteopathic contribution, eventually rendering it unrecognizable. The medical profession's contention is that if osteopaths will not or cannot justify themselves in terms of pathology, or other accepted diagnostic criteria, there is no point in pursuing the matter; they have ruled themselves out of court. But why, in that case, Korr asks, has the profession recently accepted acupuncture?

> Was there a sudden breakthrough in our knowledge of the mechanisms underlying the practice of acupuncture? Did last year see the publication of a large-scale double-blind study demonstrating the efficacy of acupuncture on thousands of patients and in dozens of disease and clinical situations? No. A practice long rejected as unproved, unscientific and unorthodox suddenly became acceptable because a few distinguished figures in American medicine visited the People's Republic of China, made some first-hand observations of acupuncture in practice, and returned to report, 'We have seen acupuncture, and it works'.

Osteopathic manipulation, Korr goes on to maintain, is not a technique which can be evaluated, like a drug, by objective criteria. It is a complex transaction between people, in the course of which 'two persons are physically, physiologically and even psychologically linked in a cybernetic loop in which each responds continually to the other's responses'; and it depends for its efficacy 'on an infinite variety of adaptations to the unique and continually changing requirements to the individual'. In a healthy person, Korr feels, a spinal lesion simply represents 'a channel of increased vulnerability' – like a fuse wire; 'whether or not disease develops depends on other factors in that person and in his life – inherited, developmental, emotional, social, nutritional, traumatic, microbial and others'.

CHIROPRACTIC

There is now little point in trying to make fine distinctions between the osteopath and the chiropractor. Significantly, if an osteopath is asked what the differences are, he will almost invariably describe certain theories or techniques which chiropractors *used* to advocate, perhaps half a century ago. A chiropractor, asked the same question, will also describe what osteopaths *used* to advocate in those days. Most osteopaths use some chiropractic ideas, and *vice versa*. Many osteopaths and chiropractors freely admit, at least in private, that though they may have begun by accepting the teachings of one school or another, experience has made them pragmatic. They continue to call themselves by the one name or the other only because it happens to represent the one in which they qualified.

Five propositions may be considered basic to chiropractic, according to C. W. Weiant and S. Goldschmidt in their book describing the ideological struggle between chiropractic and orthodoxy.

1 Subluxations, in the sense of either joint fixations or displacement slightly beyond the range of joint movement, commonly occur.

2 Subluxations are capable of provoking multiple, adverse, functional and structural changes, not only in their immediate vicinity but, by way of nervous influences in remote tissues and organs of the body, and such changes may constitute the basis of symptoms . . .

3 Postural defects may in similar fashion be productive of symptoms and may themselves be effects of subluxation.

4 Subluxations and many postural defects may be corrected manually.

5 The correction of such structural defects is followed by the disappearance of symptoms.

Substitute 'lesion' for subluxation and there is nothing in these five propositions to which an osteopath could not subscribe; so it is ordinarily on issues such as the techniques of manipulation that differences are stressed. As André Mahé put it in his *Colonne Vertébrale, Arbre de vie*, the chiropractor employs what are known as specific thrusts, or direct techniques:

the actual thrust is of short amplitude, high velocity and of minimal force, and demands great precision in terms of placing the adjusting hand, the timing and the direction of the thrust itself. Osteopathic techniques differ considerably from those of chiropractic inasmuch as they are indirect instead of direct. The osteopath employs the principle of the lever in his corrective movements . . .

Where there is a subluxation, the chiropractor traditionally thinks in terms of applying thrust to it of a particular kind; the osteopath thinks in terms of freeing it by twisting the body, using the patient's arm (or whatever provides leverage) to obtain the same result. But even this distinction appears to be dying.

The chiropractor in America, and in Britain

In the United States, chiropractic has been following a very similar course to osteopathy. Since the battles of the years between the wars, it has gradually established itself, State by State, until there are estimated to be 30,000 practising chiropractors. In the process, they too have been becoming more and more like general practitioners; and their training colleges have come more and more to resemble medical schools. The syllabus, for example, takes in nearly 1,000 hours of physiology and anatomy; 500 hours of bacteriology. The only important medical items omitted are pharmacology and surgery. As with the osteopaths, too, battles have been fought within chiropractic between the 'straights', who feel that the spine and only the spine should be treated, and the 'mixers', who accept that other types of treatment may be indicated; this, coupled with personality differences, has led to divisions. But it has not prevented chiropractic from establishing itself as a recognized therapeutic method in almost all States.

The chiropractor is ordinarily styled 'Dr', and can sign death certificates and insurance benefit certificates. Many firms employ chiropractors, and they are particularly involved in sport, notably with the Olympics teams. Recently, The National Institute of Neurological and Communicative Disorders has awarded a two million dollar grant for research into chiropractic. It is clearly well on the way to respectability – even if it rates only the briefest mention in the 1975 edition of the *Encyclopaedia Britannica*.

This change of status, however, makes it difficult to think of chiropractors any longer in terms of their original ideas and practices – as has been shown in the report of an investigation by a team from the University of Utah, designed to compare the effects of treatment by chiropractors and by doctors. As such trials go, these days, it was rather haphazard; the investigators simply went to patients and asked how they had fared, and as the patients had not been selected and matched beforehand there could be no certainty that the samples were evenly distributed between doctors and chiropractors (both of whom, inevitably, would claim they had had the more difficult cases). Nevertheless the results were instructive: there was no significant difference.

If this was a little disappointing to the chiropractors, it was humiliating to the doctors, as their line had been that chiropractic was humbug. And from the point of view of, say, an insurance company it was a powerful recommendation to accept chiropractic, which was considerably less expensive. But what also emerged from the study was that the chiropractors were no longer relying on manipulation. They did not prescribe drugs or surgery, but otherwise they used much the same conventional aids, such as heat treatment and even corsets, as doctors. It could therefore hardly be described as a trial of chiropractic; certainly not of manipulative therapy.

In Britain chiropractors, dealing as they do predominantly with bad backs, have been more faithful to the Palmer tradition. But there are still very few of them, only around a hundred – though the numbers are now growing as a result of graduations from the Anglo-European College of Chiropractic established 10 years ago.

In one respect, at least, chiropractic in Britain is better documented than osteopathy. A survey was carried out during 1973–4 in an attempt to find out how it operated, with the help of questionnaires sent out to about 50 practitioners and 300 patients, and the replies, along with 3000 case histories – though obviously they cannot be taken as a representative sample – provide a good deal of information on the subject. They show, for example, that chiropractors are mostly young, and predominantly male; and that their patients tend to be middle aged and middle class, who have suffered either from backache or neck pain for three months or more – few people, in other words, go to a chiropractor right away, if they are in trouble. Most patients have previously tried other forms of treatment, without success.

Although chiropractors use palpation, diagnostic aids like radiology have been almost universally adopted. Treatment remains 'mostly manual, and directed at the spinal column'. But the figures for how many patients benefited, how much, and how soon, can hardly be accepted as a trustworthy sample, being derived from the individual chiropractor's notes rather than from any detached study. Still, as with osteopaths, the increasing demand which chiropractors in general report for their services is an indication that their service is giving more satisfaction than what is obtainable free on the NHS.

ORTHODOXY VERSUS THE LAY MANIPULATORS

Why, then, has the medical profession not tried to come to terms with osteopaths and chiropractors? In the past it has been able to say, or at least imply, that it would, if they were willing to become one of the professions supplementary to medicine, like the physiotherapists. But when, recently, the British chiropractors took soundings with the Council which runs the Register of these professions, the Council told them that they would not be acceptable; and though it is not required to furnish reasons, the explanation is obvious.

The medical Establishment knows it has ultimate control over physiotherapists, in that no physiotherapist on the Register can accept patients except through a doctor. The chiropractors would certainly have pointed out that dentists are allowed to accept patients off the street; and as the training course at the Anglo-European College of Chiropractic compares favourably in duration and efficiency with that of medical schools, as well as schools of dentistry, it would be hard to dispute the chiropractors' case for the same rights. But if they were let in on this basis, the physiotherapists would immediately demand their independence – as, indeed, some of them already mean to do; and the whole structure of control by the profession would disintegrate. The members of the Register of Osteopaths assume that the disintegration is happening now; when invited to consider becoming one of the 'supplementaries' they declined, reasoning that they will soon be able to secure State recognition on better terms than the medical profession has hitherto been prepared to concede.

To recapitulate: the arguments put up by orthodoxy against acceptance of osteopathy and chiropractic fall into five main categories:

1 That their history shows them to have been prone to egregious diagnostic errors.

2 That there is as yet no acceptable proof that spinal manipulation is a more effective method of treating backache than the conservative way.

3 Even if it is conceded that manipulation may be effective for backache, they spoil their case by making excessive and even crazy claims for its effectiveness in treating other disorders.

4 Whether or not their methods are effective, they represent a danger to the public because they have not undergone a sufficiently comprehensive medical training.

5 Even if it were to be granted that they have a case for recognition, they cannot expect it to be conceded until they have put their house in order, by settling their differences and introducing a more unified system of training and agreed qualifications.

The medical profession's objections to the acceptances of osteopathy and chiropractic have been most cogently, and most frequently, expressed by James Cyriax – the protagonist of medical manipulation has been, paradoxically, the scourge of lay manipulators. From the time he first began to preach his own heresy in the medical journals, thirty years ago, he has rarely missed the opportunity to take side-swipes at them. His assumption has evidently been that his colleagues in the profession will be impressed by his thesis that as manipulation works, it must be wrested from unreliable hands and entrusted the general practitioners and trained physiotherapists. So far, all that he has managed to do has been to nourish the suspicion doctors have of manipulation. If its record is so tarnished, they feel, there must be something wrong with it, whether practised by osteopaths or doctors.

Long before Cyriax went into action, though, medical writers were doing their best to show that the lay manipulators had forfeited any claim to be taken seriously; chiefly because of the absurdity of their theories. For a start, there was the bone-setter with his homily to his patient that when he hears a 'pop', or a 'click', this means that the displaced bones which have been the cause of his pain are back in place again. A first year medical student would know this was rubbish! As for the idea that backache is caused by a 'nipped' nerve, it was simply anatomically impossible. The whole basis of the 'osteopathic lesion', in fact, or the 'chiropractic subluxation' was fantasy: such a thing cannot, and does not, happen!

The lay manipulator's diagnoses confirmed

The mockery of the osteopathic lesion continued until the mid-1930s. What is the lesion? – Hill and Clegg asked in their *What is Osteopathy?* 'It presses, and it does not press. It is swollen, and it is contracted. It can be demonstrated by x-ray and it cannot be so demonstrated.' The whole notion, they complained, was 'as elusive as the philosopher's stone'; all it did was to provide consolation to sufferers with something tangible, 'even though it be a straw'. Hill and Clegg did not realize it, but the slipped disk was just about to turn the laugh on their own profession. Here it was: a spinal lesion. True, it was not quite what the osteopaths or chiropractors had claimed – though in fact it had been the medical osteopath Edgar Cyriax who first advanced the disk as a possible source of pain. But demonstrably it was a lesion: and this was precisely what the orthopedists had scoffed at for so long.

It was tempting for osteopaths and chiropractors to jump on the diskwagon: but most of them resisted the temptation. They accepted that disks might prolapse; but they did not accept that this was the cause of more than a small fraction of backache cases. Most now share Irvin Korr's view that more subtle influences than disk fragments or herniated pulp are ordinarily responsible for back pain. The spinal column, he points out, contains not only the nerves, their roots and their sheaths, but also quantities of fat, connective tissues, blood vessels, and so on; and as it is known that it takes only very slight localized pressure or displacement to affect the nerve cells, it may be by this means, rather than anything so violent as a pinch, that the disturbance, and the pain, are caused. And here again, the indications are that the osteopaths have been right, and the profession wrong, in their estimate of the disk's importance.

Research into prolapsed disk has also shown that the early osteopaths and chiropractors were correct in their belief that the cause of back pain can be a 'nipped' nerve. Such was the derision poured on this idea – because it was considered anatomically impossible for the vertebrae to become displaced, short of dislocation, in such a way as to pinch a nerve – that it had been largely abandoned; but the prolapsed disk, it is now recognized, can and does do the pinching. Admittedly it can be claimed that the osteopaths were right for the wrong reasons; but at least they were right; the orthopedists were wrong. And such has been the resulting confusion within the profession that what Hill and Clegg wrote about the osteopath's lesion is wonderfully apposite to the orthopedist's disk: 'It presses, and it does not press. It is swollen, and it is contracted. It can be demonstrated by x-ray, and it cannot be so demonstrated'. And certainly it can also be said that the slipped disk has been used to give solace to sufferers, 'even though it be a straw'.

Another frequent source of mirth to the orthodox has been the contention of chiropractors that certain disorders in other parts of the body are related not just to the spinal column, but to particular vertebrae, particularly those in the neck. Such merriment is likely to be more restrained following recent research in Canada by C. Chan Gunn and W. E. Milbrandt of the Workers' Compensation Board of British Columbia, treating patients with 'tennis elbow'. All had been suffering for eight weeks, and half of them had been through the mill of treatments with steroids, local anesthetics, and even surgery. Wondering if the trouble might lie with the nerves which connect the elbow with the cervical spine, Gunn and Milbrandt examined their necks and found that though there had been no indications from x-rays, all of them were tender to finger pressure, and eighteen of them showed slight limitation of lateral movement of the vertebrae. With the help of traction and manipulation all but three of them recovered in an average time of less than six weeks.

The chiropractor's 'spinal subluxation', too, so long derided, is now creeping back into some respectability. Even Cyriax has conceded that a vertebra can be fixed 'in a faulty position within its range of movement', which is precisely what the chiropractors had always claimed. And although in orthodox circles subluxation has been a suspect term in connection with the spine, it now slips in from time to time; and as it is also coming back into use in textbooks in its original sense of partial displacement of limb joints, it will not be surprising to see it reinstated for the spine, too. It is unlikely, though, that any credit will be given to the chiropractors. To orthodoxy, when lay practitioners change their minds it is a reflection of their chronic instability. When doctors change their minds, it is an indication of the advance of medical knowledge.

Orthodoxy's most pungent derision, though, was directed against osteopaths for their belief that the sacro-iliac joint between the spine and the pelvis could be subluxated. Orthopedists bluntly insisted that it could not, and the fact that osteopaths believed it could was a reflection of the depths of their ignorance. Even some manipulators, like Timbrell Fisher, expressed doubt. But in 1969 Professor Duckworth of Toronto, with the help of advanced techniques, found that it was possible to stretch the ligaments binding the joint together – which meant that in theory at least, there could be subluxations; and some orthopedic physicians, notably Ronald Barbor, now accept that many of the troubles which used to be attributed to disk prolapse in reality arise from sacro-iliac ligament derangements.

Refusal of a fair trial

If, then, errors of diagnostic theory are to be regarded as an indication of untrustworthiness, orthodoxy has a far worse record than osteopathy and chiropractic. And doctors' second line of argument against lay manipulators – that there is no acceptable proof that their methods work, derived from scientific tests with satisfactory controls – can also be turned against them, as there have been no properly controlled trials on this basis.

Osteopaths and chiropractors have been prepared for years to co-operate in trials; it has been the medical profession, and the various bodies which have been set up to fund research projects, which have resisted the idea. In 1963 Philip Noel-Baker, a former Cabinet Minister and Nobel Peace Prize winner, described in a letter to *The Times* how as a young man he had suffered from pains variously described as rheumatism, neuritis or fibrositis, which had caused him constant and serious discomfort until a bone-setter had cured him. Later, when he had so ricked his back that he could hardly walk, an osteopath had set it right in a couple of treatments. Surely, he urged, the Empire Rheumatism Council (as it was then called) should study osteopathy, so that it could be given its proper place in the NHS? In a pained letter of reply the Chairman of the Council – an eminent rheumatologist – replied in effect that they did not propose to waste their resources on such an enterprise, and although there have been half-hearted attempts at an evaluation of manipulative therapy since, like the BAPM investigation, they have not attempted to test osteopathic or chiropractic methods.

The charge of extravagant claims

Orthodoxy's third contention, that osteopaths and chiropractors ruin their case by their lunatic pretensions to cure diseases other than backache, is perhaps the one most often heard at medical gatherings. From the start, this was the argument most commonly used against Still, and later Palmer; the first editorial on the subject in the *British Medical Journal*, in 1906, quoted in all seriousness the example of an osteopath who, after re-adjusting a joint, 'promised that the patient would soon begin to see with her glass eye. And she believed it'. Such tales have been assiduously circulated ever since. 'The extravagance of the osteopaths' claims', Jayson and Dixon explain in their *Rheumatism and Arthritis*, 'has led these practitioners to fall into disrepute'. Their far-fetched assertions, in Cyriax's view, 'have naturally turned scientific opinion against them (as is reasonable enough)'. Again and again, such sentiments are echoed.

Orthopedists evidently apply their own glass eyes to an examination of the record; otherwise they would have to admit that to a striking degree, Still's hypothesis that many disorders of the body can be traced to the spine has been vindicated by medical research. They forget that it was they who neglected the idea of referred pain, in relation to sciatica and fibrositis; when in 1948 Cyriax claimed that he had discovered the link, Stoddard mildly pointed out in the *British Medical Journal* that it had been standard osteopathic teaching for 70 years. Recently, too, there has been a growing acceptance of the view propounded in Schmorl's *The Human Spine in Health and Disease*, that the spine must not be considered as a separate anatomical entity but rather as a functional unit; spinal changes influence some organs directly, and others indirectly, he maintains, so that what happens elsewhere may depend on the spine's equilibrium – which is what Still taught.

When the claims of the osteopaths and chiropractors are examined in context too, they turn out to be much less outrageous than their critics assume. The case histories in such works as R. W. Puttick's *Osteopathy*, written over twenty years ago but still the best short introduction to the subject, suggest that manipulation can be effective in almost any condition, not necessarily because of a particular link between the lesion and the symptom, but simply because manipulation liberates, or rallies, the body's own healing forces 'normalizing' the blood supply. There is no way to be certain that the manipulation does the trick by shifting a fragment of disk, or freeing a subluxated joint, or removing some source of friction which is affecting the nerves. It may simply be auto-suggestion. Few osteopaths are now dogmatic on that issue. All they claim is that following manipulation, symptoms of almost any kind (except glass eyes!) may disappear.

'Orthodox training protects the public'

Orthodoxy's fourth line of argument – that lay manipulators lack the diagnostic training required to supply patients with a reasonable degree of safety – is also commonly illustrated with horror stories on a par with the 'glass eye' tale. It is rare to meet an orthopedist who does not have some scarifying recollection of patients who have come to him, after osteopaths have failed to cure them, who turn out to have cancer (it used to be TB, but that is now so rare, except in some immigrant communities, that it is less often cited).

This is a stance which Cyriax has taken up time after time, in his books and papers. The public, he claims, is protected, in the case of doctors, 'by standards of tuition and stringent qualifying examinations'. On what grounds, he asks, 'should manipulators be excused this discipline?' Coming from Cyriax, this is a strange reasoning. As a correspondent pointed out in the *British Medical Journal* in 1955, in the course of one of the sporadic controversies which invariably follow the publication of any of his manifestos, here was Cyriax insisting that manipulation must not be done by laymen, 'yet this is the very thing he does by relegating the work to physiotherapists'. It would have been useless for Cyriax to reply that they were different, because they were trained; osteopaths were by any standards far more highly trained. Nor was the contention relevant that before the physiotherapist went to work, a doctor had done the diagnosis; because doctors had done the diagnosis in the overwhelming majority of cases seen by osteopaths.

In any case – as indeed Cyriax has since continually if unwittingly, emphasized – the idea that the public is protected by the 'stringent qualifying examinations' of doctors, is, at least in relation to backache, a myth. As GPs endlessly complain, they enter practice knowing about Pott's and Paget's diseases, and perhaps even remembering the difference between spondylolisis and spondylolisthesis; but about ordinary backache they know nothing. Certainly – and again, Cyriax has himself made this abundantly clear – they do not know which cases of backache are suitable for manipulation, and which are not. Nor, for that matter, do orthopedists. And even the protective function of picking up the cases where a backache is caused by some rare disease can no longer be claimed by doctors as theirs by exclusive right. Some osteopaths and most chiropractors use x-rays as a matter of course; and they are also now better trained at their schools in this kind of diagnosis than the average GP, in his.

If lay manipulators were really the public danger that orthopedists have made them out to be, too, their mistakes would surely have been pounced upon by the press. Yet a leading article in the *General Practitioner* has recently admitted 'we have been unable to discover any authenticated case of an osteopath doing a patient harm in recent years'. Compared to the record of the neurosurgeons, with their disk operations, and the rheumatologists, with their steroids, the lay manipulators can claim to have been paragons of safety.

For and against a single organization

So far as the general public is concerned, the final argument against recognition of osteopaths and chiropractors as an integral but independent part of the National Health Service is probably the one which carries most weight. Common sense would suggest that a single organization, embracing all forms of manipulative therapy and all qualified manipulators, and designed to bring order into the confusion, is needed if the necessary confidence is to be won.

The attainment of some kind of unity is not now so remote a prospect as it was even a decade ago, when the disputes between the different groups, or castes, were still often bitter. Relations are today much less strained than they used to be; and not just between the groups, but between them and the medical profession. When the General Medical Council changed its rules to allow a doctor to send patients for treatment by non-medically-qualified practitioners, provided that he retained ultimate responsibility for their management and satisfied himself that the practitioner was capable, some osteopaths feared that the GMC was really playing a double game: if the doctor had to retain responsibility, they felt, he might be fearful of sending patients for manipulation – whereas before, he could simply divest himself of responsibility when patients went to the fringe. But most general practitioners appear to have welcomed the opportunity. Osteopaths and chiropractors have been enjoying greatly improved relations with doctors (one chiropractor in South London recently gave a party for the doctors who sent him patients: 30 turned up).

There is, however, some justifiable uneasiness among some lay manipulators about the possible effect of any move, such as a recent Private Member's Bill, to bring them into the NHS. As soon as the medical profession realizes that it is going to be defeated on this issue, it may concentrate on ensuring that the Register of osteopaths and chiropractors is limited to those who have gone through authorized training schools, and to ensuring that the authorized training schools as closely as possible resemble medical schools. But it is precisely because medical schools have failed, in relation to backache, that lay manipulation has flourished. And, just as many doctors are now coming to realize that the kind of training medical students get is not calculated to turn out good GPs, so many osteopaths are coming to realize that the kind of training osteopaths get is not necessarily going to turn out good manipulators. Training can ensure – at least in theory – that the manipulators who graduate will be competent. But there will still be no place for a Barker.

The osteopaths can also reasonably argue that it is the medical profession which has the more pressing need to set its house in order. So far as the public is concerned, there are two categories of doctor: the general practitioner, who fulfils a roughly similar function to a magistrates' court, dealing with simple cases and passing on the difficult ones; and the specialist. But the spine is fought over by specialties; the neurosurgeons, the orthopedists, and the rheumatologists. The neurosurgeons regard themselves, and are regarded, as the élite of the profession. They work on the most important, and in some ways the most difficult, organ of all: the human brain, and its channels of communication. By contrast the orthopedists and the rheumatologists are journeymen: bone-and-muscle setters. As things stand a rheumatologist usually sees patients referred from a GP; if he can do nothing for them, he may pass them on to an orthopedic surgeon, who may in turn send him on to a neurosurgeon; and the neurosurgeon inevitably tends to become contemptuous of the lower order.

The divisions within orthodoxy itself

The strained relations between the orthopedists and neurosurgeons were broadly hinted at in a 1967 *Lancet* survey of the attitudes of orthopedists and neurosurgeons to prolapsed disks and their treatment. With the help of a questionnaire, David Le Vay elicited that they tend to live in different worlds. 'Communication between the two surgical groups was poor, except at a small number of regional and university centres'; and there was some ill-feeling. An eminent orthopedist wrote in his reply to the questionnaire 'it is well-known that neurological surgeons over-operate for discs'; an equally eminent neurosurgeon commented 'many orthopedic surgeons do not know how to deal with disc lesions; most neurosurgeons are better equipped to deal with them'. These two attitudes, as Le Vay observed, can be regarded as complementary; but they are also disturbing. The neurosurgeon rarely knows anything about the patients' backgrounds and circumstances, because they are at two removes – GP and orthopedist – from him (sometimes three, with a rheumatologist). And after the operation, the patients often revert to the care of the orthopedist or the GP. The neurosurgeon consequently does not see, as do the others, 'frequent recurrence, root irritation, impaired back function, and disability'. The orthopedist sees 'perhaps more plainly than the neurosurgeon, that the relief of pain by technically satisfactory removal of a space-occupying lesion is not identical with social and economic rehabilitation; that there are problems of work and compensation'.

But the real problem is not so much the intrusion of the neurosurgeon, with his highly-skilled but last-resort operations; it is the resistance of the orthopedists and – to a lesser extent – rheumatologists to the introduction of manipulative and other types of therapy. Cyriax, admittedly, has suggested that orthopedists need not bother to learn how to manipulate spines; they should concentrate on their work on bone and muscle in other parts of the body, and leave it to trained physiotherapists to do whatever spinal manipulations may be indicated. But, as nobody should know better than Cyriax, this is precisely what the orthopedists have always refused to do. They have been able to accept the physiotherapist in a subordinate capacity because he is not really *treating* patients, any more than nurses do: he is merely, they believe, making their pain easier to bear. But manipulation is another matter. On the evidence, there is little hope of manipulation being taught in medical schools so long as orthopedists and rheumatologists are in control in the teaching hospitals.

Among general practitioners there is a much greater readiness to accept osteopaths and chiropractors; not surprisingly, as the most recent estimate, published in the journal *Rheumatism and Rehabilitation*, suggests that as many patients go to them, as go to Rheumatism Clinics. The authors, epidemiologists from the University of Manchester, conclude that 'as long as the orthodox and the heterodox remain in competition rather than collaboration, the main people who miss out are the patients'; and a patient who has been subjected to orthodoxy's methods is apt to be angry if a quack fixes his back in seconds. But GPs have little say in affairs of state. The medical Establishment seems certain to argue that there should be no change in the status of osteopathy and chiropractic until the report of the Working Group on Back Pain, headed by Professor Cochrane, is published; and then, it will argue that the results must be awaited of trials – which the Report will surely recommend

– of different methods of treatment; trials which could last for years.

One other possibility remains, though: that the laws relating to 'alternative medicine', as it has come to be described, will be changed by international agreement through the EEC. It is obviously illogical that in France the practice of osteopathy by laymen should be illegal – osteopaths are from time to time still charged with breaking the law, though as a rule they are given only nominal fines – when they are free to practise in neighbouring countries. Recently a campaign has opened to win recognition that Common Market law can override the laws of individual member states, in alternative as well as in orthodox medicine. An International Federation of Practitioners of Natural Therapeutics has also come into existence to lobby for recognition of the rights of such practitioners. Physiotherapists, too, spurred on by the example of the Australian G. D. Maitland, whose work on manipulation has achieved international recognition, have been growing restless, and rebel groups have been forming. It will not be easy to maintain the *status quo* until the controlled trials have been completed.

4 Postural Therapies

Certain forms of treatment for backache fit into the category 'postural'. They are of considerable diversity, but they all derive from the assumption that there is nothing fundamentally wrong with the design of the human backbone and its appendages; it is simply that through such causes as accident, illness or misuse we have subjected it to unnecessary or intolerable strain. Poor posture, as H. W. Meyerding and G. A. Pollock of the Mayo Clinic put it in 1947,

> whether it is the result of bad habits or the result of an organic defect, if maintained for a long time will result in structural changes, lessened muscular tone and pulmonary inefficiency. Impaired oxygenization of the tissues and still further lowering of muscular tone will establish a vicious circle, the results of which are lowered resistance to disease, predisposition to the occurrence of scoliosis, anemia, ill-health and chronic backache. The importance of correcting minor faults in body mechanics in their early stages cannot be over-emphasized

– a point of view which naturally was enthusiastically endorsed by the osteopaths and chiropractors, when they saw it, and remains broadly acceptable to orthodox and heterodox alike.

There is one good piece of evidence in favour of the idea that faulty posture lies at the root of most backache and related disorders: that fact that they have become a serious problem only in civilized communities, and only over the last century. Sciatica is referred to in the Paston letters, dating from the 15th century, and later in Shakespeare; but lumbago only makes its appearance at the end of the 17th century, and is not often heard of in the 18th. Perhaps the best indication that backache is a comparatively recent problem, though, is that the orthopedic text books which appeared in the mid-19th century – such as the *Manual of Orthopedic Surgery* which won the Boylston Prize for Henry J. Bigelow, later to be Professor of Surgery at Harvard – show that although the specialty of orthopedics was no longer concerned exclusively with children, it was still almost exclusively devoted to the remedying of deformities and the reduction of dislocations. Backache was not mentioned. To some extent this may have been because people still took bad backs to apothecaries and bone-setters; but back pain would surely have featured more in the medical literature of the time, and in literature in general, had it been widespread – as, for example, gout did.

It seems reasonable, then, to relate the spread of backache to the changes wrought in society by the industrial revolution. It meant that millions of children grew up in squalid slum surroundings, without fresh air and exercise, and were undernourished, so that they suffered from diseases like rickets and TB, and from spinal deformities. It meant, too, that they had to work 10 or even 12 hours a day, six days a week, tending machinery, often in unnatural postures. As they could rarely afford to go to hospital, or even to a doctor, statistics are lacking; but it seems likely that this was one of the ways in which backache began to emerge on a massive scale.

The upper and middle classes were for a while spared, as their way of life did not change so rapidly. Their problems began with the invention of the internal combustion engine. Inexorably, they began to take less and less exercise, and spend more and more of their time sitting down. As Arthur Keith noted half-a-century ago, man was well adapted to an upright posture when standing, but the fact that the whole weight of the upper part of the body was supported on the spine, he felt, must mean that the strain on the spine was greater in the sitting than in the standing position; a surmise which has recently been confirmed by research in Sweden, where backache has attracted more attention than anywhere else – perhaps because it looms large as a social problem in a country which has gone so far along the road to solving other social problems, insofar as they ever can be remedied by legislative action. Pressure on the intervertebral disks, an investigation there has demonstrated, is at its highest in the sitting position.

The value of 'postural training'

There has consequently been general agreement that one of the aims

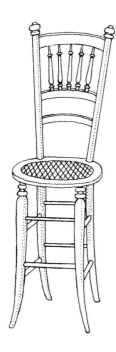

'Astley Cooper' chair
– a postural training
chair designed by a
fashionable London
surgeon in the early
19th Century to teach
children how to sit
'correctly'.

– many would insist, the primary aim – of any campaign to reduce
the incidence of backache should be to introduce or improve
preventive measures – 'physical and postural training', as Armstrong
has urged, 'especially for the young'. And there has also been general
agreement that preventive measures are effective. 'Most backache *is*
preventable', Delvin claims; 'while pain in the back can, in the great
majority of cases, be cured, you'll agree that it's an awful lot better to
stop it happening in the first place'. 'The aches and pains and misery
aren't necessary', insists the distinguished American orthopedic
surgeon, Michele: 'Many people are suffering when they do not have
to'. And most works on the subject have a section on what you should
do to avoid backache. *The trouble is that no two of them coincide.*

The disagreements over prevention policy have a long history. In
Victorian times, the recommended postural training for children
was to make them sit up straight – particularly girls as it was
considered that a stoop or any spinal deformity would spoil their
marriage chances. In 1851 a German doctor, Johann-Julius Buehr-
ing, tentatively advanced the idea that curvature of the spine in

young women might be attributable to the fashion of making them sit on backless benches, at home or at school; but this sounded so preposterous that it was ignored. In 1889, however, the young Robert Jones endorsed it, from his experience in general practice in Liverpool. 'How many of us', he wrote in a paper on the health of school children:

> having sent daughters or sisters to schools spirited and healthy, have lived to see them return round-shouldered, deformed, martyrs to headaches, pains in the limbs, or one of the many conditions which threaten to destroy their whole future happiness. This more particularly appertains to the girls than to the boys, and when we study the facts, it is not at all to be wondered at. Some years ago, a girl's life was one to be profoundly commiserated with; even now, it is not always to be envied. From the very earliest age, their instincts were checked, and artificial deportment insisted upon, as a homage to the so-called proprieties. Their natural movements were made ignorantly subservient to what was facetiously termed ladylike; but very little opportunity was given to them, and even yet there is far too little in the way of free and easy, natural, and mirthful frolic, without which every muscle in their body deteriorates . . .

Three years later, Sir James Paget (who at that time was hardly likely to have heard of Jones) expressed a similar view. Among parents' worries, he wrote, for which he was consulted,

> none is more frequent than that about lateral curvature of the spine. These fears are felt, especially, by mothers of the richer classes; and usually the fear is only for their daughters' spines. It is thought essential to the welfare of a young lady that her spine should be straight, and her form not notably unsymmetrical, and that she should habitually sit upright with her back unsupported. There is no such thought for young gentlemen, and it appears to be, chiefly, a consequence of this difference that in the well-to-do classes lateral curvature of the spine is at least twenty times more frequent in girls than in boys. For mothers seldom look at their sons' spines; and they let them sit with their elbows on the table, loll back in their chairs, and lie flat on their stomachs, and do many more such prudent things as in the daughters would be deemed shameful. Thus boy's spines grow straight; the muscles

helping to support them are not over-tired, or, when they are, they can be rested in any comfortable posture. But among girls the postures deemed graceful must be maintained until some deformity is discovered or suspected, and then the poor girls must be made miserable by the treatment deemed necessary for its cure.

There is anatomically no 'correct' spine, Paget insisted. Backache was often the result of unnecessary fears of deformity; when he investigated girls brought to him he rarely found anything the matter with them except that owing to the effort involved in sitting or standing with the body upright, 'the tired muscles ache prudently, needing rest and more various activities'. It was a mistake to think that spines should conform to an established anatomical pattern; there were probably as many varieties of healthy spines as there were of healthy chins. Even the jutting out of vertebrae, though it might look strange, no more implied that the spine was diseased than a naturally prominent nose.

Although Paget thought that the folly and mischief of making girls sit bolt upright was at last coming to be recognized – 'the good rule of letting girls grow up like boys is becoming more and more widely observed, and a larger proportion of them are well-formed, graceful and strong' – the idea that it was good for little girls, and even better for bigger girls, to sit up straight with their backs unsupported has lingered on until this day. The pamphlet *Mind Your Back*, for example, put out by the Health Education Council, is illustrated by pictures one of which shows a young man sitting slightly stooped forward over a cup of tea, with the caption 'You run the risk of back strain if your posture is bad'; and another, showing a girl sitting on a stool with her back in the best Victorian tradition, explains 'Good posture means preserving the natural shape of your backbone as closely as possible . . . Always keep your head up, your shoulders straight, and the lower part of your back hollow. You will feel better and look more attractive'. For this and other reasons, the pamphlet was dismissed as 'dreadful' in *Talk Back*, the Back Pain Association's newsletter, which quoted the comments of experts some of whom thought it useless, and others actually harmful; and whenever some expert puts forward proposals for postural training, it can be assumed that some other expert will denounce them.

Many writers, therefore, have contented themselves with advocating postural training without specifying what this training should consist of. 'Most people in this country don't pay enough attention to posture, which is why so many of us slop about round-shouldered and slouching', Delvin comments, and goes on to warn that 'if children aren't taught correct posture, they very often develop slight curvatures of the spine or tilting of the pelvis – and these malpositions can easily lead to severe back trouble later on'. But on how the correct posture should be taught, Delvin remains discreetly uncommunicative, except to remark that 'much of the success of Yoga practitioners in dealing with backache has been due to their ability to show people that they are standing badly, and to get them to hold themselves correctly'.

If sitting upright is so bad for a growing girl's spine, it is sometimes asked, how can it be that yogi do not suffer from backache? On the contrary, many people who have suffered from backache, and have taken up yoga, suffer no longer. The most likely explanation is simply that those who take up yoga do so of their own will. To ask a child to sit still, with a straight back, for any length of time against its inclination is to impose a form of torture: whereas anybody practising yoga is ordinarily free to break off, if and when mind or body rebels.

Exercises – helpful or harmful?

The other preventive panacea for backache, exercise, has a similarly erratic track record. It was only in the course of the first world war, when conscription was introduced to provide man-power for the front, that the authorities in Britain were aroused to the damage done by earlier neglect of social services, reflected in the high proportion of men who could not be accepted for active service because they were suffering from disorders ranging from flat feet to tuberculosis of the spine. And after the war, Robert Jones was successful in keeping the public alive to the need to ensure that children, at least, ought to be given adequate opportunities to enjoy fresh air and exercise. In the forces, and later in schools – even those in which games were already compulsory – physical training was introduced; and later, it became a stand-by in magazine articles devoted to fitness in general and weight-reducing in particular – and more recently, to staving off heart attacks. As a result morning exercises have become for many citizens a ritual almost as demanding as morning prayer used to be in Christian households.

But there is hardly one of the recommended exercises which has not, at one time or another, been condemned as unwise – notably 'physical training', army style. Robert Jones, a fresh air fiend, was not well disposed to the gymnasium; but where there was no alternative, he urged that attention should be concentrated on rhythmic exercises with a musical accompaniment, 'for nothing is more dreary than the old fashioned drill-sergeant's method, which had not in it one element of harmony or poetry of movement'. Referring to one of the stand-bys of PT, touching the toes with the legs straight, Mennell claimed he had cured many a case of inveterate backache by the three words, 'give it up'. And recently a campaign has begun which amounts virtually to a repudiation of most of what old-style PT stood for, at least so far as anybody at risk from backache is concerned.

Reproduced courtesy of the London Evening Standard

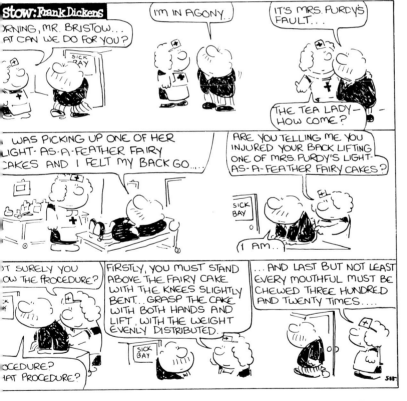

How far it has gone can be gauged from Michele's *You don't have to ache*; and as he writes as Director of Orthopedic Surgery in no fewer than five New York hospitals, and Honorary Police Surgeon to the city, in addition to his holding of the Chair of orthopedic surgery at the New York Medical College, Michele can hardly be dismissed as a purveyor of heresy. If you exercise regularly, he warns, you may think it is making you fit, but you may often be doing yourself harm – particularly if you are one of the three out of ten who are liable to back trouble; and he lists exercises which you should avoid:

> Do not touch your toes standing with your legs straight
> Do not do press-ups and pull-ups
> Do not do sit-ups unless you use a curling motion with your feet free and your knees lightly flexed
> Do not lie face down while raising the arms and legs and arching the back
> Do not lie flat on your back and raise both legs while keeping your knees straight
> Do not climb ropes or ladders, or work on parallel bars
> Do not lift weights
> Do not work with pulleys or steel springs to increase arm and chest muscles
> Do not jump hurdles
> Do not wrestle

Apart from the last two, all the exercises Michele disapproves of have at one time or another been recommended 'to strengthen the back', and a glance through the standard works on backache, where they deal with prevention at all, commonly reveals advocacy of one or more of them.

Backache and seat design

There is not even agreement over what should be avoided, to escape backache. The common belief that people doing jobs involving lifting or carrying objects are more at risk than the rest of the community has not been confirmed in a survey carried out by Yale epidemiologists; the only factors common to the group studies, described as acute lumbar disk cases, were car driving, a sedentary occupation, a suburban home, and previous full-term pregnancies.

That the way we sit is likely to be a significant risk factor is generally assumed: the trouble is that there has been no agreement

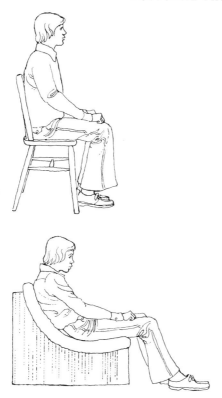

Illustrations like the above are commonly provided to contrast correct with incorrect chair design; but of much greater importance is to select and sit in chairs which happen to suit your particular needs.

on what sitting position is safest. Again and again, chairs have been designed, produced, and promoted as preventing back trouble; only to run into a barrage of criticism.

A Copenhagen surgeon, for example, Dr Aage Christen Mandal, has recently invented one with a tilting seat which, he claims, spares the typist her usual problems of stressed spine, hunched shoulders and pressure on the thighs. But when the magazine *Design* offered it for comment to Joan Ward of Loughborough University, she replied that it actually contravened the three basic principles upon which chair design should be based: that the sitter should be able to change her posture; that the lumbar spine needs adequate support; and that the main weight of the body should be borne by the 'ischial tuberosities' – the protuberances of the bottom of the spine on which we ordinarily sit. If the seat of a Mandal chair were tilted forward, she pointed out, the typist would have to brace herself against the floor or the desk; if backward, she would not be in a working position. In any case, no experimental data had been presented to show what advantage the Mandal chair offered; and they certainly would be required by education authorities, 'as the cost of purchase and maintenance of adjustable furniture is known to be extremely high'.

For a time there were high hopes that the new science of ergonomics, by which strains and stresses of the human frame were to be measured, would come up with acceptable answers. According to Paul Branton, a consultant ergonomist writing in *Talk Back* in 1977, it has not yet done so; and 'nowhere in the field of back-pain prevention is there greater confusion and speculation than in the area of seating design'. Principles are earnestly enunciated, only to be refuted; and recommendations

> usually proceed from wrong or untenable assumptions to incomplete or unwarrantable conclusions, made for unexplained reasons and aiming at unrealistic purposes. The lack of realism is easily detectable in the somewhat moralistic tone in which recommendations are couched. The mere idea that one posture is 'right and correct' while another is 'wrong' is far removed from the reality of ordinary day-to-day sitting . . .

The commonest of untenable assumptions, in Branton's opinion, is that seats can be designed which are 'correct' for all people; because each of us has different needs. And this makes a mockery of the efforts that have been made, not only by chair designers but by well-meaning organizations ranging from British Rail to the Mermaid Theatre at Puddle Dock in London, to instal 'orthopedically acceptable' seating. Mercifully for its patrons, the Mermaid found it could not afford them.

Car seats have also come in for a great deal of attention, and criticism, from orthopedists. In Cyriax's *The Slipped Disc* there is actually an appendix by Dr Bernard Watkin giving 'car seat ratings', taking into account firmness, thigh depth, shape, height, lumbar support, and so on, with one star for bad and five for cars which in Watkin's view fulfil orthopedic requirements. Most American cars get one star; only five – two Alfa Romeo models, one BMW model, the Range Rover and the Triumph Stag – rate four; none qualifies for five. But if Branton is right, such ratings are meaningless; for, as he emphasizes, each driver has different needs. It would be more to the point for each of us to find out our personal five star rating, and to choose seats adaptable to our specifications.

Some generally accepted preventive measures

There are very few preventive maxims, in fact, which have not at one time or another been challenged. It is generally accepted that beds should not sag too much in the middle, but whether this actually causes backache does not appear to have been proved; in any case, some orthopedists argue that what is of more importance is that you

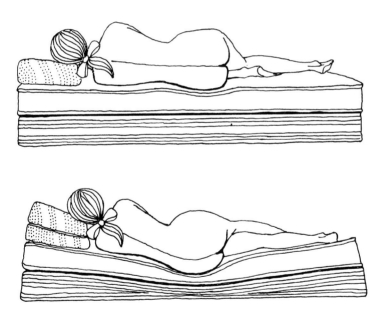

Some people find that a firm bed helps to avoid backache while a sagging bed is liable to trigger it off.

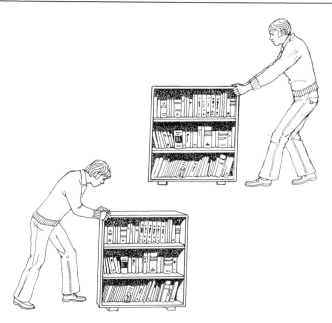

Pulling a heavy object puts less strain on the body than pushing.

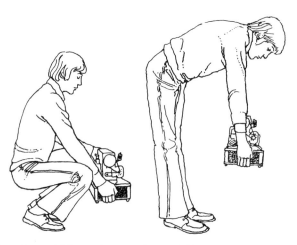

Any chore which requires stooping and lifting should be done by bending the knees and keeping the spine straight.

should never sleep in an awkward attitude (one well known London orthopedist claims that going to bed drunk is one of the common unrecognized causes of backache, because the body, doped, does not shift around to ease cramped muscles). Obesity is more certainly a risk factor; it is statistically linked to backache proneness, as to many other ills. Other things being equal, experiments have shown, pulling puts far less strain on the body than pushing, weight for weight, so pushing should be avoided when pulling is practicable. Common sense suggests that where work of any kind has to be done, it should be done in a posture which does not cause strain. In a symposium *The Lumbar Spine and Back Pain*, published in 1976, Dr John R. Glover asserts that in industry, instruction in good handling and lifting techniques is the *only* successful method of reducing the incidence of back pain; and any chore which requires stooping and effort – making a bed, say, or picking up a child – should if possible be done by bending the knees and keeping the spine straight. But in general, the golden rule – as Shaw put it – is that there are no golden rules. It is up to each individual to discover what are the precipitants of his backache, and to examine ways to avoid them, including

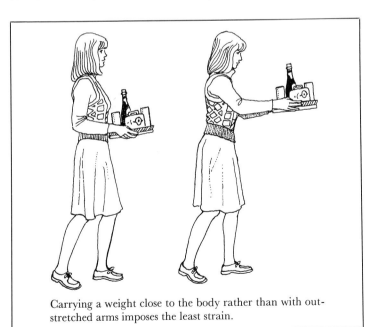

Carrying a weight close to the body rather than with out-stretched arms imposes the least strain.

exercises. A machine has recently been marketed which enables back pain sufferers to monitor their own muscle tensions, and train themselves to take avoiding action. As it costs over £200 ($380), it is unlikely to become a familiar household appliance).

SPECIFIC POSTURAL THERAPIES

Rolfing

Two maverick postural therapies remain to be considered; two of many, but deserving consideration because they have picked up an international following: 'Rolfing', and the Alexander technique.

'Bones do not hold muscles: muscles hold bones' – Stanley Lief, the man who was most responsible for establishing, or re-establishing, naturopathy in Britain used to assert; and this is a proposition which since the second world war has been adopted and expanded, originally in California, by Ida Rolf. The spine, to her, is the tentpole, and the limbs the guy ropes; but as neither can be secured to the ground, we remain upright by a balancing act, in which the muscles are the chief performers. They are remarkably good performers, given the chance; but too often an unnecessary strain is put on them by postural defects.

If, through bad habits or illness or accident or any cause, part of our bodies are out of alignment, the effect is rather similar to that of a young child's tower of bricks; as the bricks are not squared off, the higher the tower the more wobbly it becomes. In such circumstances the muscles are not free to perform their routine balancing function; they are distracted by the need to hold the whole unstable structure together. Subjected to chronic strain of this kind, they tend to lose their elasticity, and gradually we seize up – backache being one of the commonest symptoms.

'Rolfing', as it has come to be known, is based on the assumption that it is futile to concentrate on the vertebrae where the pain is felt, or even on the spine; what is needed is a breaking-down of adhesions on a massive scale from the feet upwards, so every muscle in the body can be liberated, and this requires ten sessions of 'deep manipulation'. The treatment has recently been described by Christopher Macy in *Psychology Today*. It is a sort of massage, he explains,

> except that it is not just a gentle smoothing and soothing relaxer. A Rolfer uses the points of rigid fingers, clenched fists and elbows as well as the open hand, all at high pressure, to exert the right kind

of force not on the skin but on individual muscles and groups of muscles lying deep below it in the inner cavities of the body. Sometimes, while the Rolfer is doing this, the poor tortured client has to work against the pressure, lifting an arm, say, lying on his side, while the Rolfer bears hard down on the muscles under the armpit. It *must* be good for you because it hurts like hell.

The process continues until the Rolfer can go no deeper, by which time, the theory is, all the muscles will have been stretched, all the adhesions broken down, and the body restored to its correct positioning, resembling a plumb line hanging the wrong way up – if such a thing were possible – with the head as the plumb.

Is this believable? 'If you've been Rolfed', Macy comments, 'you'll believe it because you've felt it, and observed the results'; and this is really all that can profitably be said. Many people who have been Rolfed swear by it; but it would take an unusually strong-minded individual who has been through it all to admit at the end of the tenth session that he is none the better for it. He may, too, be the better for it less because of the effect on his anatomy, than from this feeling of well-being derived from his greater flexibility. Here, at least, Ida Rolf agrees with the osteopaths, that the ultimate aim is to release and rehabilitate the imprisoned life force. The fact that we can stand or walk naturally in the posture which best suits us, releasing all our muscles to perform their proper duties, gives a psychological boost, restoring self-confidence, and sometimes rousing the individual to escape from the dead-end job, or whatever it is that had bowed him down with care.

The Alexander Principle

The basis of the Alexander technique is that instead of looking for the causes of symptoms in something wrong with the body – instead of attributing backache to slipped disks or subluxations – we should look at the way we are using our bodies, and our minds. Use, he insisted, affects functioning; and he devoted his long life to demonstrating how, with considerable success, and trying to explain how, with less success.

Alexander described how he came by the idea clearly enough in his *The Use of the Self* (1932). Growing up in Australia, he became passionately fond of Shakespeare; and after some success as an amateur reciter, he decided to turn professional – such recitations, in those days, could still attract audiences. For a while the venture went well; but after a few years he began to have throat trouble, and problems with his vocal chords. Doctors and voice-trainers could do nothing for him; and so bad did his hoarseness become that it was obviously going to wreck his career. Yet the doctors assured him there was nothing organically the matter with him. He was assumed to be a victim of what, at that time, was called 'clergyman's throat', regarded as a functional disorder brought on by too much preaching in public.

But why, in that case, did the hoarseness only manifest itself when he was performing? Could it be that he was using his voice differently, then? Performing in front of a mirror, he found that he was; 'I saw that as soon as I started to recite, I tended to pull back the head, depress the larynx, and suck in breath through the mouth in such a way as to produce a gasping sound'. There was nothing the matter with his vocal organs, it was the way he was using them that was responsible for giving the trouble; and in particular, the way in which he was using his spine, pulling back his head. This in turn, he came to realize, was related to his way of using what he described as 'the whole torso'. What he must do, he decided, was liberate the whole torso from the shackles imposed by wrong use. But this was not, he found to his chagrin, simply a matter of doing what came naturally. For what came naturally was often derived from habit – and the habit might be wrong. The torso needed not just liberation but re-education.

It is at this point, when he tries to describe the re-education process, that Alexander becomes difficult to follow – as he admitted. In the preface to a new edition of his book he remarked that what had troubled many readers was 'how to do it'; some of them had written to complain because they had been unable to teach themselves from his instructions. They must surely be aware, he had replied, 'that in spite of all the textbooks on the subjects, many people are unable to teach themselves to drive a car, play golf, or ski'; they consequently should not be surprised if they were unable to apply his technique, particularly as some of them clearly had not grasped what he was getting at; they were tending to be checked by the fact that something they did, on his instructions, 'felt wrong' whereas it was precisely what 'felt right' that they might have to get rid of, as a bad habit which had led them into error.

It is difficult, as it often is in such cases, to decide how far

Alexander was genuinely unable to explain his technique, for the same kind of reasons as his contemporary Barker: and how far he was employing deliberate obscurity in order to keep his hold on the training of his system. 'I called him a genius, and I still see no reason to go back on this', his disciple Dr Wilfred Barlow – Consultant Rheumatologist at Wembley Hospital, London – has written; 'unfortunately, Alexander was also something of a rogue'. But rogue or no—and Barlow stresses that it was not knavery; Alexander was a joker – his principle has attracted the support of several eminent men, including Aldous Huxley; and Huxley confirmed from his own experience that no verbal description could 'do justice to a technique which involves the changing, by a long process of instruction on the part of the teacher and of active co-operation on that of the pupil, of an individual's sensory experiences. One cannot describe the experience of seeing the color red. Similarly, one cannot describe the much more complex experience of improved physical co-ordination.'

Alexander was not concerned with backache as such. To him, it was simply one of the symptoms of misuse. But he was deeply concerned with one section of the spine, where the upper back is connected to the neck; the area of the body in which Alexander first detected fundamental misuse. The early chiropractors had felt much the same way, but they had relied on manipulation to deal with derangements: Alexander felt this was futile, as the derangements, if that was what they were, were the result of faulty use. The diagnosis 'slipped disk', he felt, or 'lumbago' ought often really to be 'misuse'.

The Alexander Principle, therefore, is in dispute not only with orthopedics and osteopathy, but also with ergonomy. As Barlow explains, ergonomics has sought to fit man to the machine by redesigning the machine to fit man: chairs, beds, desks and so on have been designed to lessen the fatigue and strain imposed by unnecessary movement in faulty positions. But 'the working man still arrives home fatigued'. Pain in the back affects most of the population, often with crippling severity; '75 per cent of our dentists develop troublesome back pain, over 80 per cent of our secretaries develop headaches – they have not been helped very much by better designed equipment. It is their USE which needs redesigning'.

Although the importance of use has been conceded by a few authorities – in his article on ergonomics and seats, Paul Branton describes how he had originally assumed that the wisdom of the body

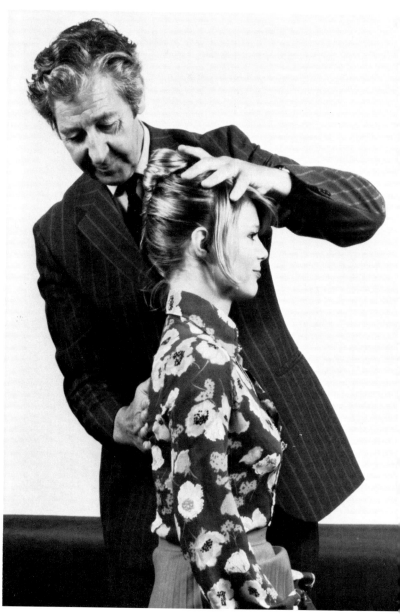

The Alexander Technique 'gives us all the things we have been looking for in a system of physical education', wrote Aldous Huxley.
Courtesy, The Alexander Institute/Arrow Books

could be trusted not to allow us to sit in harmful postures; 'now after years of systematic behavioural observation, I am no longer so sure' – the Alexander Principle has not been accepted by orthodoxy. 'Contrary to everything you may have been told before, bad posture is a disorder of the musculo-skeletal system'. Michele insists: '*Bad posture is not a bad habit*'. The Principle is, in fact, contrary to much of what both orthodox orthopedists and manipulators stand for. But for that reason, it presents a valuable alternative possibility for anybody who has found other methods of no avail; particularly if you are willing to accept that it may be faulty attitudes, emotional and mental as well as physical, which need correction.

It is no accident that many of the eminent men who have testified to the Principle's value have been searchers after ways to expand consciousness: John Dewey, Bernard Shaw, Archbishop Temple, as well as Aldous Huxley. In *Ends and Means* Huxley wrote of the Principle that 'it gives us all the things we have been looking for in a system of physical education; relief from strain due to maladjustment, and consequent improvement in physical and mental health; increased consciousness of the physical means employed to gain the ends proposed by the will and along with this a general heightening of consciousness at all levels'. And recently, the Alexander method has been praised by the zoologist and Nobel Prizewinner Professor Nicolaas Tinbergen, who is critical of the medical profession for its reluctance to accept it: 'although there are many wonderful physicians, the medical profession is an arrogant profession which thinks it has a higher place in society, which is nonsense', he has asserted. 'That attitude, linked with medical training, which is usually a generation behind, and in this case a little more, creates a lack of openness to new ideas.'

5 Acupuncture

Twenty years ago, if anybody had suggested that you should try acupuncture for your backache, you would probably never have heard of it; and if you had, you would have pointed out that it was difficult enough to move about at home without contemplating flying out to Singapore or Pekin. Acupuncture was, in fact, being practised nearer home, in Chinatowns all over Europe and the United States; but it had not taken a hold outside Chinese communities except to a limited extent in France, where it had filtered through from Indo-China.

The method used was based on an ancient Chinese tradition that the life forces, Yin and Yang, operate through channels, or 'meridians'; if for some reason the balance is disturbed, the body's equilibrium is upset, and illness results. The symptoms, though, do not necessarily indicate the real nature of the disorder. To find which organ – heart, liver, glands – is giving the trouble, practitioners sometimes perform a pulse diagnosis much more elaborate than the one normal in Western medicine, amounting almost to a qualitative 'feel' for signs. From what the pulse indicates, they know where to insert fine needles, at specific points on the meridians, which start up the flow once more, and in doing so remove the symptoms.

In the mysterious way these things often happen, the news began to circulate in Britain in the early 1960s that acupuncture could do wonders for people with rheumatism; and when a women's magazine published an account of it, some ten thousand letters came in from readers, most of them wanting to know where they could obtain it. At that time, only a handful of British doctors knew how to use it; and one of them, Felix Mann, began to train others in London. But as Mann refused to allow anybody but a qualified doctor to enrol as one of his students, the massive demand could not be met except by people outside the profession, some of them already practising nature cure and manipulation; others picked it up from books or from hastily improvised training courses; and to this day, doctors who are acupuncturists remain a small minority.

In the United States acupuncture did not enjoy the same boom. A search through the directories in New York in 1964 revealed only a single professional acupuncturist. But in 1971, James Reston of the *New York Times* had to have his appendix removed while he was on a visit to China; and although when he was operated on the normal pain-killing injections were used, he suffered afterwards from post-operative pain. Offered acupuncture, he courageously accepted. As he described it in the *Times*, the doctor

> inserted three long, thin needles into the outer part of my right elbow and below my knees, and manipulated them in order to stimulate the intestine and relieve the pressure and distension of the stomach. That sent ripples of pain racing through my limbs and, at least, had the effect of diverting my attention from the distress in my stomach. Meanwhile, Dr Li lit two pieces of a herb called *ai*, which looked like the burning stumps of a broken cheap cigar, and held them close to my abdomen while occasionally twirling the needles into action. All this took about twenty minutes, during which I remember thinking that it was rather a complicated way to get rid of gas on the stomach, but there was a noticeable relaxation of the pressure and distension within an hour and no recurrence of the problem thereafter . . .

If it had been anybody but Reston, the story would probably have been dismissed as fantasy; certainly it would have attracted little attention. And it was easy enough to dismiss the relief of his pain as coincidental. But Chairman Mao, who placed great faith in acupuncture, seized the unexpected opportunity. The China Medical Association invited two of America's most eminent doctors, Paul Dudley White and E. Grey Dimond, to China, where they examined Chinese medicine in general, and acupuncture in particular; and they reported that acupuncture anesthesia was extensively used not just to remove post-operative pain, but as an anesthetic during even the most serious operations. It worked, they were assured by the doctors (and witnessed for themselves), in the great majority of cases – though it might not work if the patient was very tense or frightened, and a general anesthetic would then be used instead. And its effects could be used even in the most protracted of operations, such as the removal of a brain tumor, which had taken six hours. The pain-killing effect, too, might last many hours after the operation.

Significantly, some of the surgeons they watched had been initially trained in Western methods. One of them, Dimond recalled, said that 'he, and practically every Western-trained physician that he knew, had been thoroughly sceptical of acupuncture anesthesia and had thought it was essentially a hoax. It was only after repeated clinical experiences that he became convinced'. And it was only after visits by further teams of doctors, some accompanied by TV and film camera teams, that Western doctors reluctantly allowed themselves to be convinced, too. 'By now', *Science* had to concede on August 18 1972, 'the scarcely veiled thought that acupuncture is some kind of a hoax has lifted, and most Western scientists who have had contact with men who constitute the closest thing available to an authority on the subject are convinced that acupuncture works – in China. The question is – Why?'

Science would have been nearer to the mark if its question had been, 'How?' The medical profession is not averse to the use of techniques for which no scientific explanation has been found provided they seem to work; but it likes them at least to appear to fit into established medical concepts. Acupuncture did not. The forces 'Yin' and 'Yang' could not be traced, nor could the meridians through which they were supposed to flow; and though there was soon a gadget on the market supposedly capable of picking out the precise points on the skin into which the needles had to be inserted, many acupuncturists doubted its validity. And so there began a search for a theory which would account for the pain-killing capacity of acupuncture in terms acceptable to Western science; a search which still continues.

How does it 'work'?

One problem has been that the nature of pain is so imperfectly understood. The ancients thought of it simply as the reverse of pleasure; not as a sensation in its own right. Then in 1794 Erasmus Darwin suggested that pain was the consequence of any excessive stimulus; warmth and coolness being pleasurable, for example; extremes of cold or heat painful. Half-a-century later, however, physiologists claimed to have discovered evidence which suggested that this was not the explanation: pain, it was now claimed, had its

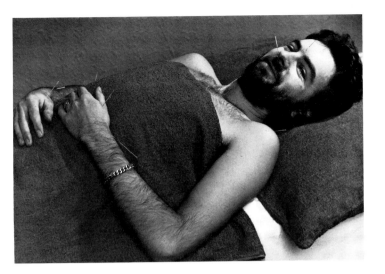

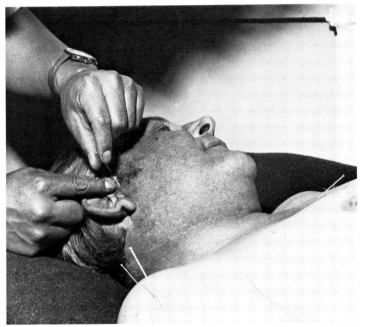

Two patients receiving treatment for backache, the needles being positioned at so-called acupuncture points. Acupuncturists claim a remarkable record of success in the treatment of back pain. Various theories have been put forward by Western doctors as to how the method 'works'.
Courtesy, British Acupuncture Association and Register Limited

own specific channels, separate from those which communicated, say, warmth; and this has since come to be accepted. But though it explains the way in which pain is felt, it does not explain why pain is sometimes *not* felt, when it ought to be. If there is anything the matter with a back, or a tooth, or any other organ, the level of pain should presumably be related to the severity of the injury, or decay. But pain in fact often comes and goes, for no apparent reason. Clearly attention has something to do with it: if our attention is sufficiently distracted we cease to feel pain, or at least to be aware of feeling it. But this does not account for the remission of pain at times when there is no distraction, and no other discernible reasons why our backs should not continue to ache.

Is there, then, some highly subjective element in pain – and, presumably, in pain-killing? Many doctors, particularly in Britain, began to favour the idea that acupuncture anesthesia works through some psychological process. The Chinese people, the common implication was, are predominantly simple-minded peasants, who have let themselves be persuaded that acupuncture will kill pain; and perhaps also because they are peasants they have a higher pain threshold, making them better able to bear it, they benefit from a kind of generalized placebo-effect, or mass auto-suggestion. 'It's probably a form of hypnosis', Alan Gilston, anesthetist at the National Heart Hospital, surmised in 1972, at the time when it was ceasing to be possible to dismiss acupuncture as nonsense; and this came to be considered the most acceptable explanation – or the least unacceptable.

Hypnosis had been largely ignored by the profession, and it might have been embarrassing to have to admit that lay hypnotherapists, who had been denounced as charlatans trading on the public's credulity, had all along been justified in their belief in its therapeutic potential. But from long experience the profession manages these somersaults without suffering humiliation; without, indeed, seeming to be aware it is making them. Besides, it was possible to contend that by placing acupuncture firmly in the hypnosis category, it might be possible to dismiss it as irrelevant for British purposes.

An attempt was, in fact, made to do just this in the Annual Report of the Medical Research Council for 1974–5. Basing its findings on an investigation by four doctors who had visited China, the Report pooh-poohed the notion that acupuncture played a significant therapeutic role even *in* China. Only about 15 per cent of patients there, it claimed, responded to it; they required three days of intensive and expensive preparation in hospital before they could be operated on with acupuncture anesthesia; and its use involved uncertainties which would be unacceptable in Western hospitals. At the same time, the rumors began to circulate that controlled trials were proving that though acupuncture worked, it worked only by placebo effect. The needles could be stuck in more or less at random.

The 'gates of pain' – a possible explanation?

There was, however, an alternative proposition. Ronald Melzack of McGill University in Montreal and Professor Patrick Wall had put forward their theory of 'gate control' of pain in *Science* in 1965. The transmission of pain signals from the parts of the body to the brain, they suggested operates through a series of 'gates' in the spinal cord. If the appropriate gate can be closed, the pain signals from the part of the body being operated upon cannot reach the brain; and the gates can be closed by a process which has long been recognized in folklore and history whereby pain is reduced or removed by 'counter-irritation' – such as a very low or very high temperature, or a fluid which causes blistering. Some counter-irritation methods have lingered on in common use, such as the application of ice to the forehead to relieve a hangover; and although no scientific explanation has been found, the assumption is that some mechanism like distraction of attention must be involved.

Working on the hypothesis that the function of acupuncture needles may be to act as counter-irritants, Melzack and his colleagues began to investigate the parallel phenomena of 'trigger spots' which are often found in cases of referred pain, and where it is known that counter-irritation can be effective in treatment. He discovered that the location of known common trigger spots broadly coincided with the points on the acupuncture charts – some of the charts several millennia old – showing where needles should be inserted for the relief of pain. It followed, if this hypothesis was correct, that perforation of the skin by needles should not be necessary: an electric current directed at the same spot should have a similar effect. And so it proved, in tests on patients with various pains, including backache.

This close correlation between trigger spots and acupuncture points, Melzack pointed out, is remarkable, 'since the distributions of both types of point are historically derived from such different concepts of medicine' – acupuncture points being traditionally related to an 'anatomically non-existent system of meridians', whereas trigger spots are 'firmly established in the anatomy of the neural and muscular systems'. But as both trigger spots and acupuncture points are associated with similar kinds of pain, and as treatment of the pain by counter-irritation works with both, it was reasonable, Melzack felt, to suppose that although they had been discovered independently and labelled differently, they 'represent the same phenomenon'.

Research to test this hypothesis has since been carried out at McGill University by Melzack and Elisabeth Fox on 12 patients suffering from low back pain. All of them had a long history of pain – six had already had disks removed by surgery; and all had failed to respond to conservative treatment. They were treated both with acupuncture and with transcutaneous electrical stimulation using an electrode, the degree of pain relief being measured by the formulae which have evolved for registering pain intensity. Both acupuncture and electrical stimulation produced pain relief estimated at more than 33 per cent in about two thirds of the patients; most of them benefited for several hours, some for days. Neither method, Melzack and Fox admitted, can be described as a 'cure': most patients need repeated treatments. But

> when it is recalled that many of the patients in this study had suffered pain for years, and several had undergone major surgery without relief, the value of a technique which brings partial relief for a few hours or days at a time is especially evident. It makes the difference between unbearable and bearable pain, between a sedentary, sometimes bedridden life and one that, for at least several hours or days a week, allows a normal social, family or business life. Even a few hours or days of pain at tolerable levels permits some of these patients to live with more dignity and self-assurance so that life in general becomes more bearable.

In the course of the trials Melzack had also satisfied himself that neither acupuncture nor electrical stimulation worked by placebo (dummy) effect or hypnosis. It was not difficult to insert needles or apply electrical stimulation in places where there was no trigger spot or acupuncture point, and to show that then, the simulated treatment did not work. And this has since been confirmed by other tests, notably one conducted recently at the Broussais hospital in

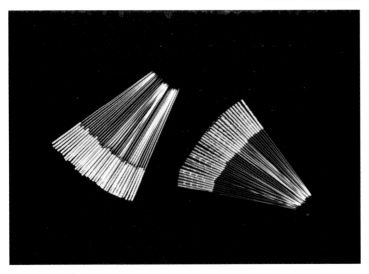

A selection of needles used in acupuncture.
Courtesy, British Acupuncture Association and Register Limited

Paris. Volunteers who wanted to give up cigarettes were divided into two groups, one given real, the other simulated, acupuncture. The results showed a significantly higher proportion of those treated by acupuncture were able to stop smoking – for a while, at least; the effects were striking over the initial six weeks, but there was a distinct falling away by the end of six months.

If Melzack's results are more fully confirmed by further research elsewhere, much will be explained which has hitherto been baffling. The fact that the Chinese, who used simply to stick in needles and leave them in the skin for a time, have recently switched over to twiddling the needles, and to passing a mild electrical current through them, becomes intelligible; they too have been moving away from the metaphysical towards the physical. The possibility also opens up of a new kind of do-it-yourself acupuncture. If electrical stimulation works as well, there is no reason in theory why patients should not be able, under supervision, to apply their own electrodes to the surface of the skin, whereas inserting needles to the correct place to the correct depth, and twiddling them, would be difficult; in some cases anatomically impossible, except for a contortionist. And Melzack's results indicate that there is no significant difference between the two, whichever method is used. Acupuncture, though, takes a shorter time – three minutes, whereas electrical stimulation takes thirty; and the anesthetic effects of acupuncture, for some reason, are on balance much more enduring: so it still appears to hold the balance of advantage.

Acupuncture's success with backache

Other theories have been put forward to account for acupuncture's effects. The discovery that the brain and the pituitary gland can make endorphins, substances which act like morphine, has prompted the idea – following experiments at the University of Virginia – that the stimulation of the needles in some way prompts nerve cells to produce endorphins in greater quantity (or of greater potency), and that this has the same result as an injection of the drug. But whether this or the gate theory or a compound of both is the answer is of less concern to you, looking for relief, than whether acupuncture will give it. And among its practitioners, there is general agreement that it works particularly well for backache and associated disorders.

In a paper on its possibilities for general practice, Elizabeth Ferris – medallist in diving at the Rome Olympics, and a qualified doctor who practises in London – has noted that in her experience, the conditions which respond best 'include those recalcitrant painful ones such as low backache, stiff painful joints, muscular aches and pains in the neck and limbs, migraine etc.' The most striking feature, in many cases, is the immediacy of the relief, graphically described by one patient as making him feel 'as if a balloon full of treacle had been pricked, and was slowly oozing out'; and though the relief is rarely complete after the first treatment, after a course as many as two out of three sufferers are free from back pain.

How does this come about? Dr Ferris is not prepared to be dogmatic about the theory; but in practice, she finds, during acupuncture the spinal muscles which have been hard to the touch as if in spasm, begin to soften, as if by some reflex action. And she goes on to make the same point as Melzack, that it works for many patients who have been fruitlessly through the orthodox mill, with drugs, physiotherapy, local hydrocortisone injections – and even, in some cases, visits to psychiatric clinics, because their doctors, unable to find any pathological cause, have assumed they must be neurotic. But she does not dispute that their backache can be psychosomatic –

the symptom of the patients' unconscious choice, to get out of an unwelcome situation, or to compensate for his dissatisfaction with his job or his home. In such cases, acupuncture can provide only temporary relief; the patient will come back for more treatment, or go off, disgruntled. But sometimes, it seems to hit the spot in a more lasting sense; though how this comes about, through physiological or psychological forces or both, has yet to be discovered.

In America Stanley Weiss, a former surgeon practising acupuncture in Florida, has recently reported a trial he has made using a combination of traditional Chinese acupuncture and counter-irritation on 50 patients with chronic low back pain which had resisted orthodox treatment – on average, they had suffered for five years; acupuncture gave complete relief to half of them, and only three reported no benefit. The effects, Weiss warned in his paper on the subject in the New York *Medical Times*, are not lasting: the treatment has to be repeated. But the improvement, he has found, is cumulative; the patients do not acquire tolerance to the needles, as they may do to drugs. And in the great majority of cases, the needling causes no discomfort.

As with manipulation, many people would prefer to go to a qualified doctor for acupuncture; but very few doctors can give it. In the US, where regulations vary State by State, it is difficult to gauge the progress acupuncture is making outside the profession; where it cannot legally be practised, estimates are unreliable. And in Britain, where anybody can set up as an acupuncturist, they are unreliable for another reason. When acupuncture first became popular a central body with a training school, the British Acupuncture Association and Register Ltd, was established; and it has tried to maintain itself in that role. But there have been internal conflicts; partly over principles, partly over personalities. On a TV programme in 1976, Sidney Rose-Neil, the dominant figure in the Association, claimed that it was the only college of acupuncture in Britain; but the claim was promptly disputed by Jack Worsley, who had split off from the Association to form a College of Chinese Acupuncture; and also by another contender, the International College of Oriental Medicine. Again, as with osteopathy, the qualifications displayed by acupuncturists means little. Personal recommendations are the safer guide.

6 Mind over Matter

You will have been unlucky if, among the friends and acquaintances who have called to see you or spoken to you on the telephone while you have been nursing your bad back, no one has been able to recommend a good osteopath or acupuncturist. You will, though, have been lucky, if no one has ventured to suggest that your pain is psychosomatic. If somebody has, your irritation will doubtless have been all the greater because you will have been in no condition to throw him out of the house. On reflection, though, you may be willing to concede – to yourself if not to your tormentor – that he could be right; or at least, that other people's backaches sometimes seem to be a neurotic symptom.

Until the Renaissance, it was taken for granted that there was, or could be, a psychological or psychic element in illness. But as the existence of an unconscious segment of the psyche had not been recognized, the assumption had been that the forces operating to cause or cure illness were external – either divine or diabolic. With the spread of rationalism and materialism, however, belief in such 'possession' began to wane, and the educated classes began to accept that the causes of illness, though indeed external, were physical or chemical – even if it remained in doubt what those causes might be. But this presented doctors with a problem, whenever they came across causes where a cure was clearly effected by non-physical means.

Two such cases, both of backache, attracted the notice of Benjamin Rush – one of the signatories to the Declaration of Independence, Physician-General to Washington's forces, and a prolific commentator on medical matters. Rush recalled how the captain of a British man of war, lying in his cabin, had leapt to his feet on hearing the cry of 'Fire', and only later realized that he was cured; and how a householder was similarly, and permanently, cured when the window of his room was accidentally smashed, and he jumped out of bed in his fright. 'I well know that toothaches, headaches, hiccoughs, etc are often removed by the sudden impression of fear', the sceptical Rush remarked; but

> to see the whole system in a moment, as it were, undergo a perfect and entire change, and the most inveterate and incurable disease radically expelled, is surely a very singular and marvellous event. If an old man languishing under disease and infirmity had *died* of mere fright, nobody would have been surprised at it; but that he should be absolutely cured, and his constitution renovated by it, is a most extraordinary fact, which, while I am compelled to believe by unexceptionable evidence, I am totally at a loss to account for . . .

In the early part of the 19th century an explanation evolved. Patients of the kind Rush had described had not really been ill: they had been victims of hysteria. This, too, presented a problem; hysteria, as its derivation from the Greek implied, was a disorder of the uterus, and consequently should only have affected women. But it was well known that in the great outbreaks of epidemic hysteria in the middle ages, such as the Dancing Mania – convulsive dancing of an involuntary nature that broke out in the streets and churches in many parts of Europe, lasting for several weeks at a time – men had often been caught up as well. The presumption was that some physical cause would be found. In the case of the 'Tarantella' outbreaks in Italy, in fact, a culprit had been named: the bite of the Tarantula spider.

Hysteria – 'a cloak for ignorance'

For a time, hysteria served as a kind of blanket diagnosis for disorders of the kind which doctors now call psychogenic – those, that is, that are considered to have originated in emotional conflict. The implication was that the mind of the patient had lost its normal control over the muscles, so that the patient either lay paralysed, or went into wild convulsions. 'Spinal irritation' – a polite medical euphemism, as patients who thought they had something the matter with them were apt to be indignant if told they were hysterical – became the standard diagnosis where no cause of paralysis or convulsions could be found; for lumbago, too; even for neuralgic

155

pain. The term 'neuralgia', Sir Benjamin Brodie remarked, merely meant that pain was 'referred' to a part of the body which was not the actual source of the pain – in this case the spine; and by far the most frequent cause, he asserted, was 'an hysterical state of constitution'. For some years, hysteria remained a respectable diagnosis – at least as far as the medical profession was concerned – particularly as it could be used to explain why unorthodox cures worked where doctors had failed. This was the reason why bone-setters, mesmerists and other quacks so often succeeded, James Paget thought, in peddling their spurious wares. 'Cold, weak, useless for want of power of will', he wrote in 1867, 'subject to all the seeming caprices of a disorderly spinal cord and too vivid a brain – a joint may be cured by the sheer audacity with which it is pulled about. If nothing in it but its portion of the nervous system is at fault, this may be cured through the influence on the mind . . . for patients love to be cured with a wonder, and the audacious confidence of all these conjurors is truly wonderful'.

By this time, however, orthodoxy was coming to be of the opinion that, as all physical disorders must have physical causes, those causes ought to be detectable; and hysteria, as a consequence, was becoming an embarrassment. In his 1875 book on back ailments J. E. Ericksen, though he had a chapter on 'spinal irritability' and its concomitants, referred or neuralgic pain, was careful to call it 'spinal anemia', the implication being that some deficiency in the blood supply was responsible; and though he did not dispute that it could lead to paralysis or convulsions he uttered a warning, destined to be the first of many, that it was a dangerous diagnosis to apply. Too often, he felt, to label symptoms hysterical served 'as a cloak for ignorance'.

At the time, Jean-Martin Charcot, professor of pathological anatomy at the University of Paris, was conducting experiments with hysterical patients in the Salpetrière Hospital; and one of the symptoms they often displayed was the 'rainbow effect', visually most striking, as the patient appeared to coil up, until lightly balanced on head and heels, her body arched like a spring. The role of the spine in hysteria had often been noted before: for example in a vivid eye-witness description of an outbreak of epidemic hysteria in Virginia earlier in the century – 'the contractions are sudden and violent, such as are denominated convulsive, being sometimes so powerful when in the muscles of the back, that the patient is thrown on the ground, where for some time his motions more resemble those of a live fish when thrown on land, than anything else to which I can compare them'. This, to Charcot, was the clue: hysteria was a neurological disorder. The mind's messages to the muscles through the spinal column were in some way being scrambled, so that they were getting the wrong instructions, or no instructions at all. And he was able to demonstrate this, to his own satisfaction, by putting hysterical patients under hypnosis – which, he assumed, was a neurological process – and showing that when hypnotized they could faithfully mimic the symptoms not only of paralysis and convulsions but of almost any kind of illness.

As it happened, Charcot's explanation of hypnosis was soon abandoned. It was easy to prove that simple suggestion could put people into the hypnotic state; in other words, that it was a psychological rather than a neurological process. And soon, it was being accepted that hysterical symptoms were the product of intervention by the unconscious mind. But so far as the medical profession was concerned, the important point was that it had been shown that hysterical symptoms were not organic; how could they be, if they were induced by a hypnotist? Hysteria could therefore be explained away as a kind of unconscious malingering, of no clinical interest, except perhaps to alienists – as psychiatrists were then called. Nobody, after all, died of backache; so if anybody were incapacitated by it, and hysteria were diagnosed, it was to an alienist that he could look for treatment. To be diagnosed by a GP as a hysteric could consequently mean banishment to the local asylum, entailing incarceration for an indefinite period, perhaps for life.

As a result, 'hysteria' came to be used only as a last resort; and by the beginning of the 20th century medical students were being taught to follow the advice of Ericksen and shun the diagnosis for fear that some real, physical cause might be missed. A. H. Tubby, whose *Treatise on Orthopedic Surgery* became a standard text book in the 1890s, was willing to accept the opinions of Paget – by this time Sir James, surgery's respected elder statesman – on the prevalence of spinal hysteria; but the chief importance of such cases, to him, lay not so much in the fact that they might not be recognized, as that more serious conditions, such as bone decay, might be classed as 'hysterical spine'.

The effects of this change can be observed to this day because, in throwing out hysteria, the profession also rejected the whole concept of the mind, or psyche, as part of the process by which diseases are caused and cured. In 1872 the London surgeon Daniel Hack Tuke had tried to separate out what we would now call the psychosomatics of the disease process from hysteria, in his *Illustrations of the Influence of the Mind upon the Body in Health and in Disease*; but he was swimming against the tidal wave of mechanistic medicine unleashed by Pasteur's work, and he was soon forgotten. Pain, the assumption now became, must have a physical cause. If no cause could be found, as so often happened in cases of back pain, the symptoms might be labelled 'functional'; but this simply implied that medical science lacked the means (or the doctor, the skill) to find the physical cause, infection or lesion.

'The flight into illness'

Shortly before the first world war a German physician, Georg Groddeck, became convinced that this new orthodox assumption was fallacious. He did not dispute that there were disease agents, such as germs; but he did not believe that they were the sole cause of diseases. He had read Freud's work, at first to deride it; but experiences with his own patients had convinced him that Freud was right – that the condition of the unconscious mind is the key to health and disease. 'In pose and posture, in attitude and in every gesture', Freud had written, 'the organism speaks a language which antedates and transcends its verbal expression.'

Groddeck, following Freud, decided that the 'It', as he described his version of the unconscious, was far more important than the Ego, which was no more than 'a mask used by the It, to hide itself from the curiosity of mankind'. The It, he felt, was the real personality: 'the deepest nature and force of man, accomplishing everything that happens with and through and in man; it is responsible for his existence, gives him all his organs and functions'. The It operated purposefully, creating health and disease: illnesses being essentially a regression to childhood, an attempt to escape from realities without suffering guilt. The 'flight into illness' gave a man the opportunity to postpone the solution of inner conflicts, sometimes to repress them so effectively that they ceased to emerge into consciousness.

But the It, Groddeck decided, also had an ingenious way of making its real meaning clear. If the symptoms were of back pain, they were telling him that there was something, or somebody, he 'could not stand' – the affected function providing the clue to the reasons for the It's intervention, much as hesitations and verbal slips were providing Freud with similar clues in psycho-analysis. And as an example – writing to Freud to elaborate on his thesis – Groddeck described how he had treated a lady suffering from so severe a pain in the region of her neck that she could not lie down on her back or her side, and had to sleep face downwards.

Could she think of any reason, he had asked her, which would have led to her punishing herself in that part of the spine? The patient eventually admitted that she could. A doctor she had been to for treatment for an arthritic arm had aroused powerful sexual excitement in her, of which she was deeply ashamed, because she assumed that such lusts were vile. Her excitement, she now recalled, and her guilty feelings, had risen when the doctor had helped her to prepare for his examination by unbuttoning the back of her blouse, which she was unable to reach herself. 'I do not remember feeling so deep a sense of shame as I had when I felt his hand on my back', she told Groddeck. 'And as far as I can judge, the painful place is exactly where his touch produced in me this strange confusion'. She went on to discuss with Groddeck the reasons for her feeling of guilt; and by the following day the inflammation on the back of her neck had disappeared. Later, her arthritis disappeared too.

Impressed by Groddeck's ideas, Freud adopted his own notion of the Id from them; and the German psychotherapist Wilhelm Reich was later also to adapt them to his purposes. Each of us has his own characteristic posture or stance, Reich contended, which represents our defences against our repressed sexuality, our 'character armour'. But this can be broken down if we are in a trance state, as under hypnosis, or in a hysterical condition; 'as self-consciousness disappears, so does the physical attitude through which a man keeps contact with the world he lives in; he loses his balance, his muscles no longer obey him, and the various relationships he has created between knowing, feeling and moving are destroyed'. And shortly before the first world war a Scots doctor, J. L. Halliday, carried the argument a stage further suggesting that fibrositis, sciatica and lumbago ought to be renamed psycho-neurotic rheumatism, because they were really a response, by certain personality types, to a situation in which they were 'suffering from unexpressed emotional tension'.

In his paper, published in the *British Medical Journal* – surprisingly, as it was rarely given to accepting work of this kind – Halliday's aim was to urge that pathology was not the only basis for diagnosis; psychopathology must also be considered, because psychological factors could bring about changes 'in chemistry, rhythm, secretion and even structure'. Doctors should not simply ask themselves, 'what has this patient got?' They must also ask, What kind of a person is he? Why did he fall ill at the time he did? Why did his illness take that particular form? Had he any purpose in falling ill? Any or all of these might give clues to the reason for the symptoms.

As examples Halliday cited case histories, including one of a shop assistant who suffered from lumbago, explaining that he felt as if he could not bend. Halliday could find nothing pathological to account for his pain, so he had tried inquiry along psychopathological lines. What kind of a man was he? He was upright – a Church Elder. Why did he fall ill when he did? He had succumbed to a suggestion that he should 'put his shirt on a horse', borrowing money to do so which he could not afford; and when he had lost it he had not dared to tell his wife. His inability to bend, Halliday suggested, was symbolic. It could be interpreted, 'I am an upright man, and do not stoop to such low pursuits as betting'; or 'I am a proud man, and cannot lower myself by telling my wife'. When this connection became clear to him, he found that he could bend quite freely.

There was also the case of a respectable man who in the heat of a political argument had struck his opponent, and been sent to prison, as a consequence of which he could not get a job: when he could not get up one morning because of back pain, the key might have been his unconscious feeling, 'I am down and out'. For other patients, the backache might be saying 'I am being spineless' in a certain situation; or 'I am not standing up to him', or 'I am getting it in the neck'. These were the kind of slangy clues doctors should be looking for, rather than concentrating exclusively on the search for organic causes; by so doing they would discover for themselves what Darwin had realized 60 years before when he said that 'the language of the emotions is of importance for the welfare of mankind'.

The 'psychosomatic' theory and backache

Halliday did not use the term psychosomatic, which had not at that time entered into currency; but it was to be popularized by Flanders Dunbar, in her *Mind and Body, Psychosomatic Medicine*, published in New York in 1947. In it she explored the idea that people catch the kind of illness to which, as personality types, they are prone.

Unluckily her ideas led to a confusion about the meaning of the term which still persists; for as colloquially employed, it commonly carries the implication – indeed, the stigma – that the symptoms are induced by the mind alone, which in turn often carries the further implication that they are not 'real', and would go away if the patient would snap out of it. But physical symptoms which are not 'real' should be classified as hysteria, and those which are 'real', but are induced by the mind (like a blush) as psychogenic; leaving psychosomatic to perform its proper function of describing symptoms which arise from an interaction of mind and body.

That this is not simply an academic distinction was illustrated in a lecture delivered to the Royal College of Physicians in 1952 by Dr R. R. Bomford, Physician to the London Hospital, on 'Changing Concepts of Health and Disease'. As a medical student, Bomford recalled, he had never even heard the term psychosomatic; and when he heard it, he took it to mean simply that a disordered mind could cause physical disease, a proposition rejected by orthodoxy, which held that organic disease would ultimately yield up all its secrets to physics, chemistry and bacteriology. And this was still the orthodox view at the time he was giving his lecture, as he was able to illustrate by quoting from the recognized authorities, such as Sir George Pickering, who had just dismissed the psychosomatic hypothesis as unworthy even of consideration by medical science.

Bomford, however, had become interested in the subject; and he felt he could most effectively illustrate why by citing his personal experience. He had himself suffered for many years from backache, which had originally been attributed to fibrositis and later to focal sepsis (fortunately for him, no site of sepsis could be found). Eventually an x-ray appeared to disclose, as he thought, the real reason: a prolapsed disk. This, he felt, could be attributed to an exhibition he had been fond of giving in his army days: a 'neck roll', which involved diving over some object, turning a somersault on a cushion, and landing on his feet again. Doing this for the amusement of the officers mess on party nights, he thought, he must have strained his back, the slipped disk and the pain being the consequence.

On reflection, however, Bomford had come to see that this was too glib an explanation. Why, if the disk was the cause, did the pain only come on from time to time? It might, of course, occur only when he had just been putting some undue strain on it; and he found that its onset did tend to follow if he 'slumped' in an armchair, or a car seat.

But why had he slumped, when it was not his normal habit to slump? Because, he realized, slumping was for him the physical expression of certain feelings. 'What we call the cause of illness', he concluded,

> is never strictly the whole cause, though it may be a necessary factor in causation in the sense that one would not have had that particular illness without that particular factor. I would not have had the particular kind of pain in my back if I had not had a protrusion of an intervertebral disc. But the protrusion of the disc was simply one link in a chain of causation.

Bomford's lecture is still, a quarter of a century later, the shrewdest brief exposition of the psychosomatic theory in relation to backache. The main reason why orthodox medicine has so signally failed to come to grips with the problem is its obsession with single causes, still being displayed in the hunt for a virus which will account for, say, arthritis and ankylosing spondylitis, and thereby rescue them from the ignominy of being classified among the disorders for which no organic explanation has been found. But even supposing that a virus *is* found, and labelled, it may avail the patient nothing, because it will not answer the question: *why* did he succumb to it, when he did? In fact it will not even answer the question, *how* did he succumb to it, because simple identification of a virus does not reveal why it should have succeeded in its depredations. Still less does it indicate what line of treatment to pursue. Of the diseases which have been re-categorized as virus-produced over the past few years, only a small majority have been rendered more treatable as a result.

Set out in Bomford's form, the psychosomatic theory is both more easily digestible than and more palatable than the common assumption, that it implies our backache is merely a symptom of some mental disturbance. If our spinal muscles are in a state of tension because of some worry, this offers a plausible explanation why they should go into a spasm, like cramp, when they are subject to a strain, even if that strain is no more severe than one they have been subjected to the day before. Here, the psychosomatic theory links up with the stress theory of disease, as put forward by Hans Selye.

The stress theory

Selye, an Austrian who went to the US in 1931, eventually became Director of the Institute of Experimental Medicine and Surgery at

162

the University of Montreal. Experimenting there with rats, he found that if he injected them with a certain dosage of an irritant, they would recover; but if he first strapped them to a board, immobilizing them, and then gave them the same dosage, they died. 'A rat wants to have his own way, just like a human being', he decided; 'I thought this kind of frustration and struggle would come about as close to the common stress situations as we can come, in rats'. From this and similar experiments, Selye confirmed his belief that it is not simply the poison, or the germ, which causes disease; it can also be the failure of the body's self-regulating mechanism, resulting from frustration or some other distracting psychological factor, which prevents us throwing off the poison's or the germ's effects.

The stress theory has proved to be a little less unpalatable to orthodoxy than the psychosomatic theory; partly because it is relatively free from Freudian associations, partly because research into stress has appeared to offer some prospect of providing quantifiable results. It may be possible, for example, to ascertain whether patients who are suffering from some disorder were subject to certain types of stress shortly before its onset – as the Glasgow psychiatrist D. M. Kissen did with TB, showing that compared to a matched group of patients with lung trouble who on diagnosis were found not to have the disease, the TB patients had had a significantly higher proportion of stressful events such as bereavement, a divorce or a broken engagement. This kind of research, however, has proved only of limited value because, as Selye emphasized, it is not the event – the 'stressor' – which is important but the individual's reaction to it. A bereavement, after all, may come as a happy release to the people involved; a divorce or broken engagement often is, to at least one of them. And attempts to investigate the possible relationship between backache and the various forms of emotional disturbance present similar problems. Following a study of nearly 1500 patients in general practice, spread over six years, Ian Gilchrist has reported finding an association between backache and anxiety; and Dr S. M. Wolkind of the London Hospital Medical College has found in his own experience that back pain patients have significantly lower levels of libido and of appetite than the normal. But, as Wolkind admits, it is difficult to decide how far this is the reason for, and how far the consequence of, their symptoms; 'the back pain may have been "caused" by an abnormal mood but, equally, the mood disorder may have been the result of chronic pain'.

Orthodoxy, therefore, still feels justified in avoiding the diagnosis 'stress', or 'psychosomatic'. It is not uncommon for writers on the subject simply to ignore the possibility that backache may be caused in part by stress. In his book for the Back Pain Association, Delvin devotes two short paragraphs to psychological back trouble, only to say that pain can be more difficult to bear if you are worried, and that if you are depressed the pain may feel worse. Crawford Adams in his textbook also gives the subject two paragraphs, under the heading *Psychogenic or Stress Disorders*; and as they reflect the attitude still prevalent in medical schools on both sides of the Atlantic, they are worth quoting. His heading, he admits, is designed

> to issue a word of warning. When the cause of a patient's symptoms remains obscure despite a thorough investigation there is a prevalent tendency – it has almost become fashionable – to discount the genuineness of the symptoms and to ascribe them to 'hysterical', 'functional', or 'psychogenic' factors, or simply to stress. This must be deplored as a dangerous policy that has led on countless occasions to the overlooking of a serious organic disease.
>
> Just because we fail to discover the cause of a particular symptom it by no means follows that the symptom is imaginary or psychogenic; it usually means only that we are not sufficiently skilled in diagnosis. Admittedly, true hysterical disorders are encountered from time to time, in orthopedic practice, but they are few and far between. Much more often a long continued organic pain leads to a distracted state of mind that is wrongly interpreted as a hysterical manifestation. It is safer to err on the side of disregarding possible psychogenic factors than to overlook an organic lesion on the supposition that the symptoms are imaginary.

There could hardly be a more forthright invitation to the medical student to cross psychosomatic factors off his diagnostic visiting list. He knows, with gratifying certainty, that he is not going to be presented with a psychosomatic case history by his examiners; and that if he cannot detect what is physically the matter with patients he will earn rather than lose credit by suggesting stress only to reject it. In the 1976 symposium *The Lumbar Spine and Back Pain* not one of the 18 sections deals with stress (except of the mechanical kind); it is mentioned in passing only in connection with theories about pain. Again, though, schools of osteopathy and chiropractic are much less dogmatic in their attitudes, devoting as they do some time to the study of psychology in relation to back pain. Irvin Korr, for example, emphasizes the importance of the history of the individual, in relation to the onset of symptoms: whether they become serious 'depends on the person we are dealing with and all the circumstances of his life, past, present and future. Here is where other unfavourable circumstances in the patient's daily life may tip the balance; here is where an abnormal stress response will tend to find the earliest and most severe expression'.

In the past few years there have been a few attempts by doctors to re-consider backache in the light of the ideas of Groddeck, Halliday, Bomford and Selye. To Harold Wolff, Professor of Neurology at Cornell, low back pain appeared to be related to a desire to carry out some action involving movement of the entire body, 'but without the actual carrying out of such activity'; for example, running away. By analogy, Wolff suggested, the muscles of a sprinter awaiting the starter's gun are tense, in a state of readiness for an effective performance; it cannot be maintained for long, but is well tolerated so long as the blank shot is eventually fired. For somebody in a state of nervous tension, however, there may be no release. The muscles may be kept in a state of tension until 'a vicious cycle ensues in which the somatic and psychic reactions to the conflict become matters of concern to the patient and further enhance and perpetuate the conflict and symptoms' – a notion which has since been elaborated upon in a paper by Frank Backus and Donald Dudley of the Veterans Administration Hospital, Seattle. Since the function of the skeletal muscles is to move the body, they argue, tension of the musculature such as that brought about by anxiety or anger 'has an early symbolic relationship with motion and activity'. If somebody finds himself in a situation where he feels the urge to, but cannot, run away, his muscles, blood and adrenalin continually hold him in readiness for action; but as no action follows, there is no release of energy to compensate for the preparation, and if this goes on long enough the whole system may break down, resulting in pain.

In *The Language of the Body* Alexander Lowen, once a student of Wilhelm Reich, argues that emotional disturbances are inevitably reflected in the condition and rigidity or flexibility of the spine – and in back pain, a complaint for which he has treated many people.

In each case, reduction of the tension in the lumbosacral muscles, mobilisation of the pelvis, analysis of the repressed conflict and a resolution of the problem of the inhibited drive results in the complete disappearance of the pain and disability. The rigidity of the backbone is not only evident in the loss of flexibility in movement, it can be palpated in the tension of the lumbar muscles.

Describing two masochists who were his patients, Lowen recalls that both lacked 'backbone'; in any situation calling for a firm stand they made an effort, but soon collapsed – a course which he has found typical in such people. He offers, though, another possible interpretation: 'the lack of a "backbone feeling" makes these individuals contract the gut to give them a sense of support; of course, it cannot, and does not, stand up; and collapse is inevitable'.

Psychosomatic treatment begins at home

What assistance – you may wonder – is all this to you, lying in bed waiting for the pain to subside? Here, Backus and Dudley offer a suggestion, discussing cases where the backache is recurrent. Sustained contraction of the musculature, originally designed to prepare us for physical activity like running, leads eventually to backache because running away is not possible; but 'when a muscular contraction occurs for the purpose of extricating a person from his current psychosocial problem, hardly ever is it utilized to solve the problem constructively'.

There have, however, been some interesting exceptions: people who have utilized their enforced leisure to work out of their system, as it were, whatever has been disturbing them, as John Robinson, Bishop of Woolwich, did when he wrote his *Honest to God* while undergoing conservative treatment for a slipped disk. And this suggests that there may be an honorable place, after all, for conservative treatment, if it is undertaken with a view to allowing the patient to work out why backache has incapacited him. Bomford's approach is relevant; he urged his fellow-members of the medical profession to study Halliday, and in particular, when confronted with a patient to remember Halliday's questions: what kind of a person is this? Why did he fall ill at this particular time? And why did he catch that particular illness? But this is something that you can do for yourself – better, in fact, than the doctor can do it for you, as you know the answers, if you have the patience and the insight necessary to track them down.

Psychosomatic treatment, then, can begin at home. What kind of a person are you? Are there certain aspects of your personality which you have repressed, or neglected, and which are now taking it out of you? Is your job, or your home life, going sour on you? If so, why? Was there any reason why your back should 'go' at the particular time it did: some cause of muscular tension, perhaps – financial, social, sexual? Why should you have got backache rather than any other ache? Can it be that it has served some purpose; releasing you from some particular obligation, or from an accumulation of worries?

Of course it can be a help if there is somebody to channel your speculations along profitable lines rather than expending them on self-pity, or self-dramatization. Ideally your doctor should be qualified to perform that function; and a few of them do. When he began to work as a London GP, Philip Hopkins came to realize that 'most patients wanted the opportunity to talk more than anything else' and given the time, they did not merely talk, they sometimes got better. The patient might present a headache, or a backache – the symptom mattered little.

> So it seemed to me that often enough the presenting symptom acts as a 'mask', an excuse with which to come to the doctor. Later I saw that the symptom was more acceptable to the patient's family and friends – and even himself – than would have been the underlying emotional causes. If the opportunity were given, the mask could be dropped.

– and the treatment lay in giving the opportunity. But few GPs have much interest in psychotherapy; and they have the excuse that even if they are, they do not have the time for it. Psychoanalysis is too costly and too protracted; psychiatrists and psychiatric social workers tend to concentrate on mental illness; and trained psychotherapists are thin on the ground. So the easiest way to explore the psychosomatic element may be to while away the hours doing it yourself. And at least the Groddeck approach affords the prospect of some wry amusement. 'What', you may ask, 'got my back up?' Or 'who is it that I want to get off my back?' – in the hope that juggling with colloquialisms may produce a flash of insight into the causes of the tension which led, when you stooped down, to your back failing to tolerate a strain of a kind it had so often tolerated before.

The comparatively new technique of biofeedback may also become a help, in promoting relaxation. Research into its use by back pain patients has been pioneered in the University of Colorado Medical Center in Denver, where a pilot study has been carried out by using devices which monitor tension rather after the fashion of the traditional lie detecting machine, by measuring either the electrical resistance of the skin, or the muscle tension itself. Some patients, it has been shown, can learn to identify the stresses which bring on their back pain – and so avoid them; or they can learn how to relieve the pain, if they are unable to avert it.

But the first need is simply to recognize that there is a psychological element in back pain: something that only a minority of sufferers accept and only a minority of doctors make allowances for. It is just as 'real' as any physical element: and it does not imply any character weakness on your part. 'The present approach to the problem', as Wolkind has written,

> accepts that in any patient with any form of illness there is a continuous two-way interaction between the patient's physical condition and his emotional and social state, and that no physical illness can be understood out of the context of the patient's mental needs, his family, and his social situation. In addition it accepts that physical symptoms occurring in the context of psychological and social upheaval can be as painful and disruptive as any caused by obvious physical pathology. With a symptom so difficult to evaluate as lower back pain, the aim should be to understand in *every patient* the contribution made by these psychological and social factors.

7 Psychic Healing, Radiesthesia, Homeopathy

Discussing the phenomenon of miraculous cures at saints' tombs in his *Illustration of the Influence of the Mind upon the Body in Health and Disease*, a century ago, the London surgeon, Daniel Hack Tuke – unlike most of his contemporaries – was willing to accept that they could be genuine; but he felt that they were not necessarily miraculous. Through the influence of expectant faith, he wrote,

> a patient, bedridden for years, is carried or manages to crawl there; the deepest emotions are stirred – hope, longing, belief – and she finds a new power in her system; an impetus is conveyed to the limbs, and she walks home with ease. Her cure kindles the faith of others, and it is not unlikely that the combined influence of her sudden recovery of the use of her limbs, and the imaginary virtues of the tomb, would restore some to health, for whom the latter alone would have been insufficient. The epidemics of cure are as definite, and admit as easily of study, as the epidemics of disease. They will also repay the labour bestowed on tracing their causes, their rise and decline and their extent.

Tuke emphasized that he was not describing cures of imaginary or hysterical symptoms, but of real disorders; and this was and is a notion which orthodoxy has been unable to stomach. Yet the evidence that there are healing forces which, for convenience, may be described as psychic is abundant, and well-attested.

Any attempt to evaluate it, though, comes up against difficulties. There is ordinarily no way in which psychic healing can be distinguished from psychological, or psychosomatic, healing: no way of deciding whether it is the intervention of the saint which promotes the cure, or the sufferer's belief in the saint's power to intervene. And as there is rarely any sure way to distinguish between

169

organic and functional symptoms, it is rarely possible to demonstrate conclusively that their removal constitutes proof of a miracle, even if it is allowed for argument's sake that miracles can happen.

SPIRITUAL HEALING

These difficulties were discussed in D. J. West's *Eleven Lourdes Miracles*. A member of the Society for Psychical Research, London, (he has since been its President) Dr West was not a sceptic in the sense of declining to accept the possibility of miraculous cures; but when he applied the standard rules of orthodox medical science to the cases, all of them accepted by the Church as miraculous, in none of them could he accept that the evidence was convincing.

The first he cited, for example, was the case of Mlle Clauzel, who in 1937 began to suffer from arthritis of the spinal vertebrae, with deformation of the bones, and bouts of intense pain. Other symptoms followed: convulsions, indigestion, and a bladder disorder. According to her doctor, the digestive troubles began to become more and more acute until loss of appetite was almost complete, and the patient took hardly any food at all; 'wasting was rapid and very considerable; her breath had a strong odour of acetone; the pulse became rapid and the pressure low'; and eventually, in 1943, her doctor said she had not long to live. But when she was carried on a stretcher to hear Mass on the Feast of the Assumption, she suddenly expressed a desire to get up, walked back to her home, lunched with a big appetite, lost all her former symptoms – and was still free from them nine months later. Examining the evidence, however, West noted that although Mlle Clauzel had suffered from her spinal disorder for six years, at no time had there been any complete investigation of her symptoms, of the kind which are routine in modern hospitals; and, significantly, the bone deformations shown on x-rays while she was ill were still there after her recovery. The symptoms, West felt – convulsions, sudden attacks of pain – pointed to hysteria as the cause. And whether or not this was the correct diagnosis, West argued, the fact that the patient's condition changed suddenly and dramatically for the better was not relevant to the main issue. 'It cannot too often be stressed', he contended,

> that in order to establish that a real organic change has taken place, there must be a change observable by x-rays or laboratory tests, or at least a definite change in the clinical signs (e.g. reflexes,

measurements, chest sounds, etc.) elicited by skilled medical examinations. In the absence of such objective evidence, no amount of change in the patient's feelings, attitude or behaviour, however dramatic it may appear to the onlooker, is sufficient to provide scientific proof of an organic cure . . .

Yet should your backache resist treatment, and lead on to convulsions, pains in various parts of the body, and rapid wasting, until your doctor thinks that you are not long for this world, if your symptoms are as suddenly and completely removed as Mlle Clauzel's it is unlikely that you will lose sleep wondering whether they were hysterical or organic. For if, as is clear, in the great majority of cases of backache doctors cannot confidently point to a cause, or decide whether the disorder is organic, the argument becomes academic. The salient feature of the Clauzel case is that her back trouble and the symptoms associated with it were suddenly and effectively banished. And as there are scores of such case histories it is eminently reasonable, if the idea appeals to you, to visit some shrine where healing miracles are being reported, or go to a healer.

Healers usually treat patients by some variant of the traditional Christian technique of the laying on of hands. Sometimes the healer lay his hands on, or close to, the patient's head; sometimes on, or close to, the region where the pain is felt. Sometimes the healer's hands appear to take over, making movements independent. Or he may use the method known as 'magnetization', the hands being drawn down from the patient's head to his feet in a stroking motion calculated, or so the practitioners believe, to draw out the baleful influences causing the pain. And many healers find they have their most gratifying successes with backs – though this may be because the straightening up of an arthritic spine, which previously had been bent over until it looked like a question mark, is obviously much more impressive to an audience, and to the patient's friends, than, say, the removal of internal symptoms. The late Harry Edwards, founder of the National Federation of Spiritual Healers, performed this feat many times at demonstrations in the Albert Hall in London, and once at least on film for a TV programme. The doctor appearing with him, in the role of resident sceptic, claimed that the straightening was accomplished by physiotherapy; but if so, it was not of a kind physiotherapists practise. Psychic force is the more plausible explanation.

But what is the psychic force? Most healers assume it is divine in origin, and consequently does not need to be explained in scientific terms. But as healers frequently report certain physical manifestations such as intense pins and needles in their fingers, during the laying on of hands, or of warmth or coolness emanating from the patient's body, the recent tendency has been to think in terms of some force comparable to magnetism, as yet undiscovered, which the healer is able to channel through to his patients. But again, you may reasonably feel, the precise nature of the force is immaterial, so long as it works for you.

Within the medical profession there is now much less antipathy to 'faith' healing (as it is still commonly called by the public, though its practitioners dislike the term) than there used to be. When the Archbishops of Canterbury and York set up a Commission in the 1950s 'to consider the theological, medical, psychological and pastoral aspects of Divine Healing', and invited the British Medical Association to assist, the BMA set up an investigation of its own; and its report in 1958 claimed that its members had seen 'no evidence that there was any special type of illness cured solely by spiritual healing which cannot be cured by medical methods which do not involve such claims', and went on to advance all the stock explanations why people had been deluded into believing in such cures: mistakes in the diagnosis of the disorder, 'spontaneous remission', coincidence, and auto-suggestion. Although these explanations are still often heard, however, they are rarely so dogmatically expressed as they were 20 years ago, chiefly because there is much less confidence now than there was then that medical science has, or soon will have, all the necessary answers.

In 1977 the National Federation of Spiritual Healers was formally notified, in response to a query to the General Medical Council, that a doctor might recommend patients to have treatment from healers, provided he retained ultimate responsibility for patients' management, and satisfied himself of the healers' competence. And this, as with osteopaths and other lay practitioners, disposed of the old fear of the danger of going to a healer – that his treatment, if successful in removing the symptoms, might simply be masking their cause. So there is nothing now to prevent you from going to a healer with the blessing – or at least the permission – of a member of the medical profession.

The only warning which he can now reasonably give you against healing is that though its effect on your back may appear miraculous, such cures are not lasting. On this issue there is no satisfactory evidence, as healers do not have the funds to follow up their cases, and naturally they tend to hear later only from those patients who remain grateful for what they have done. But in view of the similar inadequacy of orthodox methods, even in the short term, it is not a very impressive line of argument; particularly as you have nothing to lose if the treatment fails – not even money, as healers do not ordinarily charge for their services, though often there will be the equivalent of a church offertory box, sometimes placed in an aggressively prominent position. Nothing may come of your visit; but you may be as lucky as the British actor Bill Maynard. During the making of his *Froggitt* TV series, which was to be no. 1 in the ratings in 1976, Maynard had disk trouble, and was instructed to sleep on a board and wear a steel corset. He still suffered agonizing pain; and in a stage production, he was reduced to performing in a wheelchair. Then, a visit to a spiritual healer in Brighton, Tom Pilgrim, worked 'like magic'; the corset was discarded and Maynard was once again able to enjoy the pleasure of a comfortable bed.

RADIESTHESIA

Another variety of psychic healing is radiesthesia, whose origins lie even further back in history. When anthropologists began to study tribal communities they found that divination was a standard procedure, both to diagnose the nature of a disorder and to select the appropriate treatment. The diagnosis was usually undertaken much as it is by some spiritualist mediums today; the witch doctor going into a trance state to acquire the information from the gods or spirits. But often, an aid would be used, such as a pendulum; its movements were believed to give the correct replies to the questions asked. And this technique – sometimes varied by the use of such alternatives as the water-diviner's hazel twig – was to be exploited early in the present century by the Abbé Mermet, who described in his *Radiesthésie* how, with the help of a pendulum, he learned to diagnose disorders more accurately than doctors could.

The pendulum is still used, in a variety of ways. Some practitioners let it swing over a chart, marked out so that the direction of the swinging 'bob' or weight indicates the nature of the disorder from which the patient is suffering, and points also to the appropriate remedy – often homeopathic, as this is commonly the method of treatment preferred by radiesthetists. Others ask the pendulum questions to which the 'bob' replies positively or negatively according to whether it swings clockwise or anti-clockwise. There is also a gadget, originally invented by the American scientist Albert Abrams, sometimes described as a 'Black Box', designed as an aid. In one type, diagnosis and treatment are obtained by a method resembling the way a violinist tunes his instrument, with the help of a sheet of rubber connected with numbered dials: the dials are rotated until the rubber becomes 'sticky' to the touch, the point at which the stickiness occurs indicating, through the number on the dial, what is the matter with the patient and what can be done for him. The Black Box has excited the particular hostility of the medical profession. Yet when a version of it was tested by Sir Thomas Horder and a committee of scientists half-a-century ago, he had to admit 'no more convincing exposition of the reality of the phenomena could reasonably be desired'.

It is not too difficult for anybody who concedes the possibility of Extra-Sensory Perception to accept the proposition that illness can be diagnosed by divination, even at a distance. It is harder, though, to accept that it can be *cured* at a distance. The explanation ordinarily given by radiesthetists is that the patient puts himself, in some unexplained fashion, in tune with the instrument – on much the same principle as Isaak Walton explained telepathy three centuries ago; that if two lutes are strung and tuned to equal pitch, and one is played upon, the other will answer with a faint but audible harmony. An alternative explanation is that the emanations are not limited by time or space – any more than telepathy is. It makes no difference whether the patient is in the room with the box, or thousands of miles away.

Reliable evidence for the effectiveness of radiesthesia in the treatment of backache is hard to come by, partly because there are no trustworthy statistics, partly because people who have been successfully treated by the method, grateful though they may be, do not necessarily wish to publicize the fact (one well-known public figure privately admits his back trouble was cleared up by a radiesthetist, but he has not cared to acknowledge the fact). Perhaps the most remarkable cure was reported by Jack Leach, Racing Correspondent of the Sunday *Observer*, in 1962. Scotch Delinquent, a promising steeplechaser, had been unwell; so a few hairs from its tail were sent to a radiesthetist, who with the aid of his instrument diagnosed that the horse was suffering from subluxated lumbar vertebrae, which he proceeded successfully to 'adjust'. Leach, however, knew of another case where the diagnosis had been incorrect; and several accounts have been published of how radiesthetists have been caught out by jokers – the most recent being one in *World Medicine*, by David Delvin (the author of *You and Your Back*). The specimen of hair which Delvin sent, purporting to be his, was in fact from his cat. The diagnosis was over-strain: Delvin magnanimously admitted that his cat 'had been a bit neurotic that past week, so perhaps he wasn't far out'.

In Britain, radiesthesia has come to be called radionics; and as a former Secretary of the Radionic Association, John Wilcox, has admitted, 'a radionic instrument alone can do nothing. It is as good as its user, and is of secondary importance. Non-physical energy can only be monitored by the human psycho-neural system'. There is as yet no way of knowing how radiesthesia/radionics works, or how often it works; but as it is hard to see how it can do any harm, it may be worth trying, if the opportunity presents itself – except in some American States, where it is illegal.

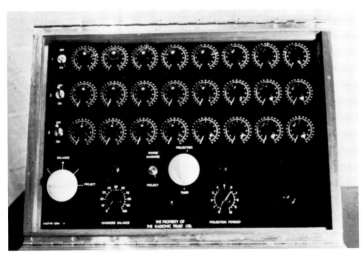

A type of instrument used by many Radionics practitioners, both for the initial analysis and for treating a wide range of conditions.
Courtesy, The Radionic Association

HOMEOPATHY

Some homeopaths will think it odd to find themselves bracketed with healers and radiesthetists; but it is now beginning to look as if their place is in the psychical, rather than the physical medicine category.

As propounded by Samuel Hahnemann in 1810, homeopathy was based on two ideas. One was of ancient lineage, having been found in tribal communities; that 'like cures like'. A fever, on this reckoning, is not a disorder; it represents the body's struggle to throw off a disorder. The right medicine, therefore, is a drug which, given to a healthy person, would produce a fever – *eg*, as quinine does.

The other principle was that decreasing the strength of a drug, so far from diminishing its effectiveness, can actually increase its potency, so that a microdose will be more effective than an orthodox full-strength dose. And these are the principles that homeopaths still apply in treatment. Back pain – like any kind of pain – is treated with a microdose of a drug which, at full strength, would cause pain.

Homeopaths, however, emphasize that it is never simply a matter of identifying the symptom, and looking up the appropriate remedy in their *Materia Medica*. It lists a great many possible drugs; which of them is prescribed, and the potency at which it is given, will depend on the homeopath's judgment of the needs of the individual patients – as distinct from their specific symptoms. It is the person who is ill; they insist, and the person who must be treated. This incidentally also keeps them more on the look-out for 'referred' pain from other parts of the body masquerading as backache – which, they claim, is very common.

There is consequently no homeopathic treatment just for back-ache; and sufferers would be ill-advised to experiment with any of the remedies unless they have the kind of knowledge of homeopathy which comes from accepting it for years as a matter of course. Even then – and this is where the psychic element comes in – the correct drug to take, and the correct potency, may be a matter of 'hunch'. And as there is no scientific explanation in orthodox terms why diluting a drug should make it more potent, the most likely hypothesis is that some element of mind-over-matter is involved. Some animals, it is known, can detect minute traces of substances, comparable to a microdose, in their diet. Perhaps we, too, have some long buried instinct which can latch on to the curative properties of a drug, even when it is present only in almost infinitesimal quantities.

8 Naturopathy, Yoga

There are some therapies which are not designed to treat backache as such, but which are claimed to set you up so that you are unlikely to suffer from it; and of these the longest-established are Nature Cure – described by its practitioners as naturopathy – and Yoga.

As its name implies, Nature Cure is based on Hippocratic principles. If you lead a healthy life – eating the right kind of food in moderation, taking adequate exercise, and so on – the theory is that you will not fall ill. With the discovery of germs and viruses, the theory appeared discredited, because for a time it seemed that although good health, by promoting better resistance, had some beneficial influence on infections in helping people to recover who would otherwise have succumbed, it would not give any protection from contracting a disease. But with the gradual elimination of many of the epidemic-type diseases, and their replacement as killers by cancer, heart attacks, and respiratory disorders, Nature Cure has been coming into its own again.

With heart attacks, in particular, it is now generally recognized that what has come to be called the psychosocial element creates the main risk factors: smoking, excessive consumption of animal fats, lack of exercise, stress. And it seems reasonably certain that back pain will eventually be found to be in the same category, though with lack of exercise and bad postural habits playing the most destructive part. Naturopaths accordingly recommend remedial exercises, along with changes of diet, as the way to avoid backache. The prescribed exercises, though, and the diet vary according to the notions of the individual naturopath. In any case, 'straight' naturopaths – in the sense of practitioners who rely entirely on preventative measures, eschewing any other kind of treatment – are now seldom to be found. Most members of the British Naturopathic and Osteopathic Association practise manipulation.

YOGA

Although not a therapy in the ordinary restricted sense of the term, Yoga provides a combination of postural and psychological exercises from which many back pain sufferers claim to have derived benefit.

In his *Yoga Against Spinal Pain*, published in 1971, Pandit Shiv Sharma provides a brief introduction to the general theory of Yoga, before going on to deal with its particular relevance to the treatment of back problems with the help of meditation, yogic postures, and breathing exercises – emphasizing that they must be considered together; 'Yoga always involves the mind with the body'. Muscle tone, he explains, is affected by mental as well as physical impulses; normally flexible muscles may become rigid owing to a worry or tension. Yoga works by, in effect, 'oiling' the various parts to 'ensure a smooth running and efficient working of the psychosomatic machine'.

Before starting, Sharma warns, it is important to realize that the *Asanas*, or yogic postures,

> are not just simple exercises but sustained, scientific patterns of posture. No jerky movements are involved and even in some dynamic *Asanas*, the movement has to be of a slow, spontaneous, uniform nature. The neuro-muscular system is so composed that for every group of muscles that go into contraction, another group undergoes relaxation. In tension states this reciprocal innervation becomes defective. *Asanas*, by their very nature, reorganize and recondition the system to bring about physiological harmony between the two

The bulk of Sharma's book is devoted to illustrations of the *Asanas*; and several of them, it has to be said, flatly contravene current orthopedic opinion, and could just as easily appear in a Back Pain handbook to illustrate the kind of exercises back pain sufferers should avoid. Confronted with this contradiction, Yoga teachers reply that the exercises are not designed to prevent, let alone to cure, back pain as such; they are carefully graded gradually to improve muscle tone until a healthy mind/body relationship is established. By the time the individual is doing the kind of exercises that orthopedists now frown on, in other words, they will not put an undue strain on his back: on the contrary, they will further strengthen it.

There are no statistics by which the effectiveness of Yoga in relation to back pain can be judged; but in any case, its teachers are in general agreement that it ought not to be embarked upon simply as a form of treatment for that or any other disorder. For those who have the patience and determination to undertake the preliminary training, to the point where they can carry on themselves, it at least offers a well-tried system for promoting relaxation, which can be resorted to at odd moments, and at no cost.

The Way Ahead

To sum up . . . We know little about the causes of backache; and it is by no means certain even if we knew more about them, and how to diagnose them, that this would be much assistance in treatment. Knowing 'more', in this context, usually refers to knowing more about the agents of disease, germs and viruses, and the processes by which they insinuate themselves; and these often reveal little or nothing which is of use in the search for ways by which the disease may be eradicated. It is as if, looking for ways to combat addiction, somebody were to discover the precise way by which alcohol, tobacco or opium create 'tolerance'. It would be a remarkable achievement, for which the researcher could expect a Nobel prize; but it would not necessarily lead to any reduction in the consumption of cigarettes, or the number of alcoholics.

Most of the research into the causes of backache has in any case been limited, because of orthodoxy's devotion to physical, or chemical, solutions. Discussing rheumatoid arthritis, for example, Crawford Adams admits that 'the cause is unknown', yet insists that 'only two possibilities deserve serious consideration: 1) that the disease is due to auto-immunity; and 2) that it is caused by infection'. But if auto-immunity is responsible – if the body's defence mechanism gets fouled up, so that we begin to make war, as it were, on our own joint linings – the question remains: why the palace revolution? And if some source of infection should be found, the question remains: why did the palace bodyguard not crush the insurgents? This kind of question is all too rarely asked; and when it is, researchers can rarely find funds to look for the answers, because the Medical Research Council and fund raising bodies like the Arthritis and Rheumatism Council, dominated by consultants brought up in the old mechanist tradition, prefer investigations whose results are quantifiable.

A typical example of the conventional approach appeared recently in a report leaked for fund-raising purposes, from St Bartholomew's Hospital, London. Scientists there, the *Sunday Times* reported, 'believe they have found the cause of most cases of osteoarthritis' – tiny crystals which have the same effect on the lubrication system between the joints, as tiny slivers of metal have on the cylinders of an internal combustion engine. The discovery, according to the report, indicated that osteoarthritis of this kind is due to 'an inborn error of metabolism', offering the prospect of a straightforward drug cure. But why should it be inborn? Might it not be an error of metabolism induced by, say, stress? It might, of course, but stress is unwelcome to researchers, in that it represents an area over which they cannot exercise any quantity control. As for the idea that the discovery of the crystals offers the prospect of a straightforward drug cure, the path medical science has taken over the past thirty years is littered with the corpses of similar expectations.

The kind of research project which secures financial backing is apt to be on the lines of one in progress at the Royal National Orthopedic Hospital into certain joint disease reactions, such as 'glucose 6 phosphate dehydrogenase, 6 phosphogluconate dehydrogenase, and NADPH oxidation (being an indication of penthouse shunt activity), lactate dehydrogenase and NADH oxidation (being an indication of glycolytic activity) and succinate dehydrogenase (being an indication of Krebs cycle activity)'. The other current fad being ergonomics – the study of the efficiency of people in their working environment – there is also a passion for research with gadgets which will produce 'objective and reproducible measurements of various static and dynamic aspects of work' – according to B. J. Sweetman in a paper on the subject – 'with the ultimate aim of seeking correlations between these factors on the one hand and the incidence of back pain on the other'. They include an 'inclinometer', to be positioned between the shoulder blades, electrical recorders of back muscle activity, and an accelerometer which can be attached to the belt to measure low back vibration. But the search for objectivity of this kind is the pursuit of an illusion, because it has to leave out such vital, but as yet not measurable, elements as emotional and social stress.

There is, admittedly, a certain amount of epidemiological research, such as a project being carried out at Guy's Hospital into what is described as the natural history of back pain; one of the aims being to try to identify possible risk factors in much the same way that some have been identified in the case of heart attacks – cigarette smoking, high blood pressure, excessive consumption of animal fats. But the immediate need is for research designed to compare the different types of treatment available; and it seems certain that this will be the chief recommendation of the Cochrane Committee investigating the treatment of back pain.

It is fortunate, therefore, that the General Medical Council's new rules have cleared the way for investigations which will allow osteopaths, acupuncturists and others to use their techniques in controlled trials. But it will not be enough for the trials to concentrate simply on comparing techniques. 'The new orthopedics is more than surgery', Sir William Osler claimed half a century ago. 'The orthopedic surgeon is a teacher, a personal teacher, and in two directions – of the patient's mind quite as much as his muscles and joints. It is not simply a surgical matter, but an individual, human problem, requiring prolonged attention and study of each case'. The weakness of today's controlled trials is that they seek to eliminate any such subjective element. They may show whether one type of manipulation gives better results than another, or whether manipulation on balance is more effective than rest and aspirin; but they will not show the extent to which, say, rapport between manipulator and patient contributes to the treatment's success. The findings of the Utah investigation by R. L. Kane and colleagues, comparing chiropractic with orthodox treatment, may have been negative, revealing no significant difference between the two, but they also showed, according to the published report, 'the powerful potential of the patient/doctor relationship in effective treatment, whether in chiropractic or in traditional medicine'. It is this potential which most needs to be realized.

The results of trials, in any case, will not be available, except perhaps in press leaks, for some years. In the meantime, if you suffer from backache there is no point in deluding yourself that the doctor – or any other practitioner – 'knows best'. You yourself know best; or at least have the capacity to know. 'Tired muscles', as Paget put it, 'ache prudently'; indications, physical and mental, are forever warning us when we are at risk and perhaps prompting us what to do to find effective treatment. The wisdom of the body may have been largely brainwashed out of us; but it can be recovered, if we can learn to liberate instinct and insight.

A Short List of Organizations

GENERAL

Back Pain Association
Grundy House
Somerset Road
Teddington
Middlesex TW11 8TD

ORTHODOX

American Medical Association
535 North Dearborn Street
Chicago
Illinois 60610

Food and Drug Administration
Department of Health, Education
   and Welfare
330 Independence Avenue
Washington D.C. 20201

National Institute of Neurological
   and Communicative Disorders
Department of Health, Education
   and Welfare
Public Health Service
Bethesda
Maryland 20014

British Medical Association
British Medical Association House
Tavistock Square
London WC1H 9JP

General Medical Council
44 Hallam Street
London W1N 6AE

Medical Research Council
20 Park Crescent
London W1N 4AL

Institute of Orthopaedics
234 Great Portland Street
London W1N 5HG

The Arthritis and Rheumatism Council
   for Research (formerly British
   Arthritis and Rheumatism Council)
Faraday House
8–10 Charing Cross Road
London WC2H 0HN

Chartered Society of Physiotherapy
14 Bedford Row
London WC1R 4ED

Institute of Orthopaedic Medicine
81 Belsize Lane
London NW3 5AU

British Association for Rheumatology
   and Rehabilitation
Royal College of Physicians
11 St Andrews Place
London NW1 4LE

MANIPULATIVE THERAPY

International Federation of Manual
   Medicine
Dr M. E. Burleigh Carson
28 Wimpole Street
London W1M 7AD

British Association of Manipulative
   Medicine
22 Wimpole Street
London W1M 7AD

OSTEOPATHY

American Osteopathic Association
212E Ohio Street
Chicago
Illinois 60611

Kirksville College of Osteopathy
and Surgery
Kirksville
Missouri 63501

American Academy of Osteopathy
2630 Airport Road
Colorado Springs
Colorado 80910

Osteopathic Medical Association
114 Wigmore Street
London W1H 9FD

British School of Osteopathy
16 Buckingham Gate
London SW1E 6LB

London College of Osteopathy
25 Dorset Square
London NW1 6QG

Society of Osteopaths
27 Leadenhall Street
London EC3A 1AA

General Council and Register of
Osteopaths
16 Buckingham Gate
London SW1E 6LB

British Osteopathic Association
8–10 Boston Place
London NW1

CHIROPRACTIC

American Chiropractic Association
2200 Grand Avenue
Des Moines
Iowa 50312

Anglo-European College of Chiroprac-
tic
Cavendish Road
Bournemouth
BH1 1RA

British Chiropractors' Association
120 Wigmore Street
London W1H 9FD

British Pro-Chiropractic Association
Sec: B. Barraclough-Fell
38 The Island
Thames Ditton
Surrey KT7 0SQ

POSTURAL THERAPIES

The Ida Rolf Foundation for Structural
Integration
PO Box 1868
Boulder
Colorado 80302

The American Center for the Alexander
Technique
142 West End Avenue
Apartment IP
New York
NY 10023

Society of Teachers of the Alexander
Technique
3 Albert Court
Kensington Gore
London SW7 2ET

The Constructive Teaching Centre
18 Lansdowne Road
Holland Park
London W11 3LL

The School of Alexander Studies
61a Onslow Gardens
London N10 3JY

ROLFING *There is no organization in the UK at
the time of going to press; there are, however, a
number of individual practitioners. See also
Naturopathy section, below.*

ACUPUNCTURE

The Center for Traditional Acupunc-
ture
American City Building
Columbia
Maryland 21044

American Society of Chinese Medicine
PO Box 555
Garden City
NY 11530

British Acupuncture Association and
Register Ltd
34 Alderney Street
London SW1V 4EU

Traditional Acupuncture Society
St Albans House
Portland Street

Royal Leamington Spa
Warwickshire CV32 5EZ
*This organization has a College
attached to it:*
College of Traditional Chinese
   Acupuncture
Registrar: M. A. C. Twigg, FCCAC
Halsway Mews
Halsway
Crowcombe, Nr Taunton
Somerset

International College of Oriental
   Medicine
Green Hedges House
Green Hedges Avenue
East Grinstead
RH19 1DZ

British Medical Acupuncture
   Association
15 Devonshire Place
London W1N 1PB

NB The British Associations keep records
of members in the United States.

PSYCHIC HEALING, RADIESTHESIA, HOMEOPATHY

American Federation of Spiritual
   Healers
Sec. R. Babine
6 Bridle Path Circle
Framingham
Massachusetts 01701

The American Center for Homeopathy
Suite 506
623 Leesburg Pike
Falls Church
Virginia 22044

RADIESTHESIA: *No official organization in
the US.*

National Federation of Spiritual Healers
The Old Manor Farm Studio
Church Street
Sunbury-on-Thames
Middlesex TW16 6RG

The Radionic Association
16a North Bar
Banbury
Oxon OX16 0TF

The Psionic Medical Society
Sec: Carl Upton
Garden Cottage
Beacon Hill Park
Hindhead
Surrey

British Homoeopathic Association
Basildon Court
27a Devonshire Street
London W1N 1RG

The Faculty of Homoeopathy
The Royal London Homoeopathic
   Hospital
Great Ormond Street
London WC1N 3HR

NATUROPATHY, YOGA

National Association of Naturopathic
   Physicians
609 Sherman Avenue
Coeur d'Alène
Idaho 83814

British Naturopathic and Osteopathic
   Association
Frazer House
6 Netherhall Gardens
London NW3 5RN

The British Wheel of Yoga
Glyn Galleries
High Street
Glyn Ceiriog
Llangollen
Clwyd
North Wales

The Community Health Foundation
188–194 Old Street
London EC1V 9BP
*This organization teaches a method of hatha
yoga and also runs classes in Rolf technique.*

The International Federation of Practitioners of Natural Therapeutics
21 Bingham Place
London W1M 3FH

Bibliography

ADAMS, J. CRAWFORD *Outline of Orthopedics* Edinburgh, 1976

ANDRY, NICOLAS *Orthopaedia* London, 1743

APLEY, A. GRAHAM (ed.) *Recent Advances in Orthopaedics* London, 1969

ARMSTRONG, J. R. *Lumbar Disc Lesions* Edinburgh, 1958

Arthritis and Rheumatism Council *Lumbar Disc Disorders: a handbook for patients* London, 1971

BACKUS, FRANK, and DONALD L. DUDLEY 'Observation of psychological factors and their relationship to organic disease' (in Lipowski, 1977)

BARBOR, RONALD 'Low backache' *British Medical Journal*, 8 Oct. 1955

BARBOR, RONALD 'Scleroscant Therapy' (unpublished)

BARKER, HERBERT *Leaves from my life* London, 1927

BARKER, L. F. and JOHN TRESCHER *Backache* Philadelphia, 1931

BARLOW, WILFRED *The Alexander Principle* London, 1975

BAUER, LOUIS *Lectures on Orthopaedic Surgery* Philadelphia, 1864

BEAUCHAMP, GUY 'Manipulation of the cervical spine' *Rheumatism*, July 1965

BECKER, ROLLIN E. 'Diagnostic Touch' *Yearbook* of the American Academy of Osteopathy, 1964

BELL, CHARLES *Operative Surgery* (2 vols) London, 1807, 1809

BELL, CHARLES *Observations on Injuries of the Spine* London, 1824

BENN, R. T. and P. H. N. WOOD 'Pain in the back' *Rheumatology and Rehabilitation*, August 1975

BIGELOW, HENRY J. *Manual of Orthopedic Surgery* Boston, 1845

BLYTHE, PETER *Stress; the modern sickness* London, 1975

BOMFORD, R. R. 'Changing concepts of health and disease' *British Medical Journal*, 21 March 1953

BOURDILLON, J. F. *Spinal Manipulation* London and New York, 1973

BREMNER, R. A. 'Manipulation in the management of chronic low backache' *Lancet*, 4 Jan. 1958

BRISTOW, W. R. 'Manipulative surgery: Sir Herbert Barker's demonstration at St Thomas's' *Lancet*, 27 Feb. 1937

BRODIE, BENJAMIN *Diseases of the Joints* London, 1850

BRYCE, ALEXANDER 'Mechano-therapy in disease' *British Medical Journal*, 3 Sept. 1910

BURNS, B. H. and R. H. YOUNG 'Protrusion of intervertebral disc' *Lancet*, 6 Oct. 1945

BURNS, B. H. and R. H. YOUNG 'Backache' *Lancet*, 10 May 1947

CARSON, H. M. BURLEIGH 'Manipulation' *General Practitioner*, 21 June 1974

186

CONSUMERS' ASSOCIATION *Avoiding Back Trouble* London, 1975

COOPER, SIR ASTLEY *A treatise on dislocations* London, 1823

CRISP, E. J. 'Damaged intervertebral disk: early diagnosis and treatment' *Lancet*, 6 Oct. 1945

CYRIAX, JAMES 'Lumbago' *Lancet*, 6 Oct. 1945

CYRIAX, JAMES 'Fibrositis' *British Medical Journal*, 31 July 1948

CYRIAX, JAMES 'Backache' *General Practitioner*, 21 June 1974

CYRIAX, JAMES *The Slipped Disc* London 1970

DELVIN, DAVID *You and your Back* London, 1975

Department of Health and Social Security *Prevention and Health: everybody's business* London, 1976

DILKE, T. F. W. *et al.* 'Extradural corticosteroid injection in management of lumbar nerve root compression' *British Medical Journal*, 16 June 1973

DIMOND, E. GREY 'Medical education and care in People's Republic of China' *Journal of the American Medical Association*, 6 Dec. 1961

DORAN, D. M. L. and D. J. NEWELL 'Manipulation in treatment of lower back pain: a multicentre study', *British Medical Journal*, 26 April 1975

DOVE, COLIN 'Osteopathy' *Nursing Times*, 29 Jan. 1976

DOVE, COLIN 'A history of the osteopathic vertebral lesion' *British Osteopathic Journal* iii, 3, 1967

DUMMER, THOMAS G. and ANDRE MAHÉ *Out on the Fringe* London, 1963

DUNBAR, FLANDERS *Mind and Body* New York, 1955

EBBETTS, JOHN 'Spinal manipulation in general practice' *Practitioner*, 1964, 192, 260–5

ERICKSEN, JOHN ERIC *On concussion of the Spine* London, 1875

FERRIS, ELIZABETH *Acupuncture* (unpublished)

FISHER, A. G. TIMBRELL *Treatment by Manipulation* London, 1948

GALTON, LAWRENCE *The Patient's Guide to Surgery* New York, 1976

GERVIS, W. H. *Orthopaedics in General Practice* London, 1958

GIBSON, T., *et al.* Chymoral in the treatment of lumbar disc prolapse' *Rheumatology and Rehabilitation*, Aug. 1975

GILCHRIST, IAIN C. 'Psychiatric and social factors related to low back pain in general practice' *Rheumatology and Rehabilitation*, May, 1976

GLOVER, J. R. *et al.* 'Back pain: a randomised trial of rotational manipulation of the trunk' *British Journal of Industrial Medicine*, 1974, xxxi, 59

GOWERS, SIR W. 'Lumbago' *British Medical Journal*, 16 Jan. 1904

GRODDECK, GEORG *The book of the It* London, 1935

GRODDECK, GEORG *The Unknown Self* London, 1937

GROSSMAN, CARL M. and SYLVIA GROSSMAN *The Wild Analyst* London, 1965

GUNN, C. CHAN and W. E. MILBRANDT 'Tennis elbow' *Canadian Medical Association Journal*, 1976 vol. 114, p. 803

HALLIDAY. J. L. 'Psychological factors in rheumatism' *British Medical Journal*, 30 Jan. 1937

HALLIDAY, J. L. 'Psychological aspects of rheumatoid arthritis' *Proceedings of the Royal Society of Medicine*, 1942

HALLIDAY, J. L. *Psychosocial Medicine*, New York, 1948

HARTFALL, S. J. 'Stress and the rheumatic disorders' *Practitioner*, Jan. 1954

HEWITT, D. and P. H. N. WOOD 'Heterodox practitioners' *Rheumatology and*

Rehabilitation, Aug. 1975

HILL, CHARLES and H. A. CLEGG *What is Osteopathy?* London, 1937

HIPPOCRATES Translated by Francis Adams London, 1939

HOLMES, T. H. and HAROLD WOLFF 'Life Situation and backache' *Psychosomatic Medicine,* 1952, xiv, 18

HOOD, WHARTON *On Bonesetting (so-called)* London and New York, 1871

HOOTON, E. A. 'An anthropologist looks at medicine' *Science,* 20 March 1936

HUXLEY, ALDOUS *Ends and Means* London, 1937

IVERSON, LARRY D. and D. KAY CLARKSON *Manual of Acute Orthopedic Therapeutics* Boston, 1977

JAYSON, MALCOLM (ed.) *The Lumbar Spine and Back Pain* London, 1976

JAYSON, MALCOLM, and ALLAN DIXON *Rheumatism and Arthritis* London, 1974

KANE, R. L. *et al.* 'Manipulating the patient: a comparison of the effectiveness of physician and chiropractic care' *Lancet,* 29 June 1974

KEITH, SIR ARTHUR 'Man's posture: its evolution and disorders' *British Medical Journal* 17, 24 March 1923

KEITH, SIR ARTHUR *The engines of the human body* London, 1925

KELLY, MICHAEL 'Steroids' *Rheumatism,* April 1965

KELSEY, JENNIFER 'An epidemiological study of acute herniated lumbar intervertebral discs' *Rheumatology and Rehabilitation,* August 1975

KEYNES, GEOFFREY *Life of Sir Astley Cooper* London, 1922

KORR, IRVIN M. 'Andrew Taylor Still Memorial Lecture' *Journal of the American Osteopathic Association,* 1974

KORR, IRVIN M. *The Physiological Basis of Osteopathic Medicine* New York, 1970

LE VAY, DAVID 'A survey of surgical management of lumbar disc prolapse' *Lancet,* 3 June 1967

LE VAY, DAVID 'British bonesetters' *History of Medicine Quarterly,* 1971

LIPOWSKI, Z. *et al. Psychosomatic Medicine: Current trends and clinical applications* New York, 1977

LOWEN, ALEXANDER *The Language of the Body* New York, 1958

McCLUSKEY, THORP *Your Health and Chiropractic* New York, 1952

MACDONALD, GEORGE, and W. HARGRAVE WILSON *The Osteopathic Lesion* London, 1932

McKIBBEN, BRIAN *Recent Advances in Orthopaedics* Edinburgh, 1975

MACY, CHRISTOPHER 'Rolfing' *Psychology Today* Nov. 1977

MAITLAND, G. D. *Vertebral Manipulation* London, 1973

MAIGNE, ROBERT *Douleurs d'Origine Vertébrale* Paris, 1968

MARSH, HOWARD 'On bonesetting' *British Medical Journal,* 7 Oct. 1882

MATHEWS, J. A. 'Symposium of lumbar intervertebral disc lesions' *Rheumatology and Rehabilitation,* Aug. 1975

MATHEWS, J. A. 'Backache' *British Medical Journal,* 12 Feb. 1977

'Medical Correspondent, A' 'Bone-setting: its history and its dangers' *Times,* 24 Feb. 1911

MELZACK, RONALD and PATRICK WALL 'Pain mechanisms: a new theory' *Science,* 19 Nov. 1965

MENNELL, JAMES *Backache* London, 1935

MEYLER, L. *Side effects of drugs* Amsterdam, 1966

MICHELE, ARTHUR A. *You don't have to ache* New York, 1971

MIXTER, W. J. and J. S. BARR 'Rupture of the intervertebral disk' *New England Journal of Medicine*, 2 Aug. 1934

MONK, C. J. F. *Orthopaedics for Undergraduates* Oxford, 1976

MOYNIHAN, BERKELEY (ed.) *The Robert Jones Birthday Volume* Oxford, 1928

MYLES, A. B. and J. R. DALY *Corticosteroid and ACTH treatment* London, 1974

NOEL-BAKER, PHILIP 'On manipulation' *Times*, 5 Feb. 1963

Osteopathic Blue Book (Forthcoming)

PAGET, JAMES *Selected Essays* London, 1902

PERKINS, GEORGE *Orthopaedics* London, 1961

PINALS, ROBERT S. and SUMNER, FRANK 'Relative efficacy of Indomethacin . . . in rheumatoid arthritis' *New England Journal of Medicine*, 2 March 1967

PUTTICK, R. W. *Osteopathy* London, 1956

RAAF, JOHN 'Some observations regarding . . . protruded lumbar intervertebral disk' *American Journal of Surgery*, April 1959

ROMER, FRANK *Modern Bonesetting for the Medical Profession* London, 1915

ROMER, FRANK, and L. E. CREASY *Bone-setting* London, 1911

SCHIOTZ, EILER, and JAMES CYRIAX *Manipulators Past and Present* London, 1975

SCHMORL, GEORG, and HERBERT JUNGHANNS *The Human Spine in Health and Disease* New York, 1971

SELYE, HANS *The Stress of Life* New York, 1956

SHELDRAKE, T. *An Essay on Causes of the Distorted Spine* London, 1790

SIGERIST, HENRY *A History of Medicine* (vol 1) New York, 1951

SMITH, AUDREY 'A survey of the osteopathic diagnostic method' *British Osteopathic Journal* 1968, iv, 1

STILL, ANDREW *Autobiography* Kirksville, Mo., 1908

STODDARD, ALAN *Manual of Osteopathic Practice* London, 1969

SWEETMAN, B. J. *et al.* 'Monitoring work factors relating to back pain' *Postgraduate Medical Journal*, 1976

THATCHER, DONALD 'One hundred cases of low back pain' *American Journal of Surgery*, April 1959

TUBBY, A. H. *A Treatise on Orthopaedic Surgery* London, 1891 (2 vols 1912)

TUKE, DANIEL HACK *Illustrations of the Influence of the Mind upon the Body in Health and in Disease* London, 1872

WATSON, FREDERICK *Hugh Owen Thomas* Oxford, 1934

WATSON, FREDERICK *Sir Robert Jones* London, 1934

WEIANT, C. W. and S. GOLDSCHMIDT *Medicine and Chiropractic* New York, 1959

WEISS, EDWARD and O. S. ENGLISH *Psychosomatic Medicine* Philadelphia, 1957

WEISS, STANLEY 'Acupuncture in low back pain' *Medical Times*, Oct. 1975

WEST, D. J. *Eleven Lourdes Miracles* London, 1957

WILSON, RALPH, and S. WILSON 'Low back-ache in industry' *British Medical Journal*, 10 Sept. 1955

WOLF, STEWART, and HAROLD WOLFF *Headaches* London, 1955

WOLFF, HAROLD *Stress and Disease* Springfield, Ill., 1968

WOLKIND, STEPHEN 'Orthopaedic aspects of sexual behaviour' *British Journal of Sexual medicine*, March 1977

WOLKIND, STEPHEN 'Psychogenic low back pain' *British Journal of Hospital Medicine*, Jan. 1976

Index

INDEX